Living in the State of Stuck

How Assistive Technology Impacts the Lives of People with Disabilities

Fourth Edition

Marcia J. Scherer, Ph.D., MPH, FACRM
Director, Institute for Matching Person & Technology

D1376146

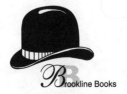

Brookline Books

ISBN 978-1571290984

Copy Editing by Suzanne Ryan
Cover design by Joyce Rooklin
Interior design and typography by Joyce Rooklin
Cover photo: *Brian and Reiko, Santa Cruz, CA 2003.* "Brian" has tetraplegia due to a spinal cord injury from a motorcycle accident in 1978, when he was 17. His story is among those featured in this book. Photo appears courtesy of Foster Andersen, Santa Cruz, CA.

Library of Congress Cataloging-In-Publication Data
    Scherer, Marcia J. (Marcia Joslyn), 1948-
        Living in the state of stuck: how technology impacts the lives of
    people with disabilities / Marcia J. Scherer. — 3rd ed.
            p. cm.
        Includes bibliographical references and index.
        ISBN _____(pbk.)
        1. Physically Handicapped — Rehabilitation — United States.
        2. Self-help devices for the disabled — United States.
        3. Technological innovations — United States. I. Title.
    HV3023.A3S34 2000
    362.4'0483 — dc30   2005-28662
                                                              CIP

BROOKLINE BOOKS
P.O. Box 1209 Brookline, Massachusetts 02445

For Orders:
BROOKLINE BOOKS
400 Bedford St.
1st Floor - SW 03
Manchester, NH 03101
1.800.666.BOOK (2665) or 603.669.7032

CONTENTS

Praise for the second edition of **LIVING IN THE STATE OF STUCK**

"In our interviews with people with spinal cord injuries, many times when we think we've heard something new, it's as if we're exploring new territory and we run up against a wall that has graffiti on it saying, 'Marcia Scherer was here.'"
—**Tom Nantais,** *Project Co-investigator, Spinal Cord Injury Peer Information Library on Technology*

"Ms. Scherer takes a very interesting and thought-provoking look at assistive technology... [T]hrough stories of people with disabilities, she illustrates the potentials and the limitations of current technology as well as the epidemic of technology abandonment.... [T]his fun and easy-to-read book is excellent for health care professionals, employers, parents, and all people with disabilities. It is an intelligent book, written for and about real people and real situations."
— *Spinal Cord Injury Life Magazine*

"I really felt the need to write and say thanks for developing such a wonderful and valuable book! Your book offered me new insight into characteristics of use and non-use. It should be mandatory reading for all special education personnel."
— **Erin Simunds,** *graduate student*

"I agree with Dr. Scherer's premise that people's perspectives and expectations will determine the success or failure of their attempts at using assistive technology... In the book, I read a lot of my own thoughts that I had when I started using my brace and my artificial legs... In conclusion, I recommend this book strongly for anyone in social work or in any field dealing with physical rehabilitation. It provides an excellent way of 'stepping into the minds' of people who have had a traumatic accident or are otherwise physically disabled."— **Peter J. Boulay,** *student*

"If you are struggling to develop a broader concept of 'outcomes' in your technology services, read this book. It provides a much needed framework for people involved with the provision of assistive technology. It will help us better understand how people with disabilities feel about the devices they use, and what are the outcomes of our interventions... It reminds us that technology is one way to maintain connection with the world, but it is only one part of the solution. She has provided an insightful forum that can and should be used to stimulate broader discussion in the field."
— **Alexandra Enders,** *Rural Institute on Disabilities University of Montana*

"Although the focus is on individuals with physical disabilities, the information in *Living in the State of Stuck* can be used easily in supporting individuals with other disabilities and their use of technology to enhance capabilities and quality of life."
— *Journal of the Association For Persons With Severe Handicaps*

"The life stories related in Scherer's book serve as crucial reminders that 'technology alone is rarely the answer to a person's enhanced quality of life.' The author presents many important questions that must be answered when recommending a device for a person... The author provides the reader with a personalized view of the world as experienced by persons with disabilities. The book presents information that would be helpful to both the seasoned professional and someone new to the rehabilitation field."
— *Journal of Rehabilitation Research and Development*

Praise for the first edition of **LIVING IN THE STATE OF STUCK**

"Marcia Scherer persuasively reminds us that as technology is used to increase ...als with disabilities to become productive members of ...ole person must be taken into account. For assistive

technology to provide the maximum benefit, services that address the emotional, personal, and social needs of the individual in adjusting to and using these devices must also be provided."
— Senator Tom Harkin, *Former Chair, Subcommittee on Disability Policy, U.S. Senate Labor and Human Relations Committee*

"Begins with a subtle exposure of some of the common psychological and functional effects of severe disabilities, then incrementally draws the reader into the complexities of disability and assistive technology use.... There is much to be gleaned by those involved in the study of social issues, as well as persons with disabilities who are trying to figure out where technology fits in their lives."
— *Disability Studies Quarterly*

"Very perceptive... looks at many rehabilitation subtleties that are often overlooked by the busy professional..."   — *JPO: Journal of Prosthetics and Orthotics*

"Provides the reader with a personalized view of the world as experienced by several persons with disabilities.... Helpful to both the seasoned professional and someone new to the rehabilitation field."
— *Journal of Rehabilitation Research and Development*

"Dr. Scherer brings an important, holistic approach to the delivery and use of assistive technologies."   — Jan Galvin, *President, Galvin Group Ltd.*

"Misdiagnosis and abandonment of assistive technologies is a national problem. Dr. Scherer gives us a consumer-driven, person-centered model to match the person to the device to get us all out of a state of stuck. It is an intelligent book about real people."— Dr. Harry J. Murphy, *Founding Director, Center on Disabilities, California State University, Northridge*

"This is a marvelous book! It is a must-read for all professionals who work with individuals with physical disabilities. Happily, it is also an easy read and a fun read.... Dr. Scherer skillfully uses the personal experiences of people with disabilities to make key points about the role of technology in people's lives. This is a caring book written for those who care."— Roberta B. Trieschmann, Ph.D., *author, Spinal Cord Injuries: Psychological, Social, and Vocational Rehabilitation*

"An interesting and thought-provoking book. Through example and discussion, accented with stories about and words directly from consumers, Dr. Scherer has been able to provide insight into both the potentials and limitations of technology, as well as the importance of its application within a general intervention/assistance program."
— Gregg Vanderheiden, Ph.D., *Past President, RESNA; Director, Trace Center*

"If you are involved, or want to be involved, in the prescription, fitting, modification, or design of assistive technology, you will learn from this book. If you are new to the field, you will gain information on spinal cord injury, cerebral palsy and a brief history of the rehabilitation process, including the independent living movement. If you have been involved in design, without dealing with the personalities of the clients, you will learn about how people with disabilities feel about assistive technology, and how their attitudes affect their acceptance of the technology."
— Peter Axelson, MSME, *Beneficial Design, Inc., Nevada*

"Marcia Scherer's gift to us in this book is that she stimulates us to ask good questions. As always, the hard part is not to answer but to ask the right questions."
— Dr. Frank G. Bowe, *Hofstra University*

Preface

by Frank Bowe

When I was the chief executive of the American Coalition of Citizens with Disabilities (ACCD), then a major Washington, DC-based umbrella lobby group, I hired a bright young woman to run our rehabilitation training programs. The best I could do to accommodate her cerebral palsy was to provide her with a keyguard to fit over her electric type-writer. A few years later, Rita Varela took a job with General Telephone & Electronics (GTE) in Florida. By that time, personal computers had become commonplace in the office. The PC — with its quick-and-easy error correction, spell-checker and function keys — liberated Rita. For the first time in her life, she was able to produce work that reflected her intelligence and knowledge. Rita quickly became an expert in computer programming. She even wrote a book in her spare time explaining how to use a PC to perform advanced mathematical functions. *Victory Over Statistics* (GTE, 1989) is impressive enough a work. What makes the book even more meaningful to me is what it represents — the fact that with technology, Rita achieved victory over the functional limitations from her cerebral palsy.

This idea — that an individual with a disability, plus the right device, can function as a person without limitations — had fascinated me for some time. It compelled me to write *Personal Computers and Special Needs* (Sybex Computer Books, 1984), the first full-length text on high technology and people with disabilities. The book's theme still strikes me. I see it in action when friends of mine who are blind or have severe learning disabilities listen to the synthesized speech produced by their PCs, rather than trying to read the screen. I see it when other friends with tetraplegia talk to their PCs, rather than type. And I see it when I and others who are deaf read on a screen what others say.

When — as is now happening — technology removes limitations, what we as individuals with disabilities can do depends strictly upon our abilities, training and experience. The devices liberate us to become what we optimally can be. At the same time, these products render vacuous any excuses we might have used before. We are forced to confront the fact that our lives will be what we make of them. We become responsible for ourselves. When we exercise that responsibility in work, in our families, and in our communities, we achieve the real meaning of independent living.

This relationship between technology and people with disabilities raises a lot of difficult questions. Marcia Scherer explores many of these issues by showing what people with disabilities do with technology — and what technology in turn does to them.

Among the questions now is that of who should pay for the new devices. The fact that someone like Rita Varela can use a PC to perform gainful employment suggests that it is in society's best interest to provide her with the devices she needs. With them, she is no burden to the taxpayer; indeed, until she died a few years ago, she paid her fair share of payroll and other taxes, helping to support others in our society.

As a subset to that question, should we link government payment for technology to an individual's commitment to, in effect, pay us back by working? That is, should no-cost technology be available only at the workplace and, by extension, at schools and job-training programs? If we answer that question affirmatively, we are limiting the "right to technology" by circumscribing it to conditions under which society realizes a return on investment.

There are arguments on all sides of these questions. One could say, for example, that someone like Rita should purchase the special aids she needs from her take-home pay. Alternatively, one could say that someone who needs technology uses it not only to work but also to live a more meaningful and rewarding life. Indeed, people with very severe disabilities may not even be employable. Tying technology to work denies such individuals any access to no-cost devices. Society should provide these people, under this argument, with technology they need regardless of whether or not they work.

To illustrate, the Television Decoder Circuitry Act of 1990 [P.L. 101-431] requires that all 13" or larger television sets sold or manufactured in the United States after July 1993 include built-in chips enabling the set to receive and display captions or subtitles. The chips themselves cost under $10 to manufacture, and are included as part of the purchase price of the set. Broadcasters, advertisers and others pay the cost of producing the captions themselves. Our nation made a national policy statement in that Act: TV is an important enough part of American society today that we should make it accessible to all of us.

The next step makes television equally accessible to individuals with blindness and low vision. The Individuals with Disabilities Education Act of 1990, P.L. 101-476, authorized demonstrations of what is called "descriptive video service," in which one audio channel of a stereo TV is used to broadcast spoken descriptions of the video action blind people cannot see. Effective since April 1, 2002, Video Description for Video Programming requires that broadcast stations and multi-channel video programming distributors provide video description.

More and more, we are finding that we can use the telecommunications infrastructure to provide important accommodations for people with disabilities. By equipping telephone company central offices and switching stations with speech synthesis, speech recognition, and other important capabilities, we can make those functions available to virtually all Americans with communication-related disabilities — at very little or even no added cost to them.

To illustrate, Title IV of the Americans with Disabilities Act of 1990 (P.L. 101-336) requires that all 1,600 telephone companies in America ensure that deaf people and others using telecommunications devices for deaf people (known for short as TTYs) have full and equal access to all telephone-based services. By July 1993, TTY users must be able to make and receive calls to and from all 50 states, 24 hours a day, 7 days a week. Title IV provides TTY users with these services at no incremental cost to them.

The Technology Related Assistance for Individuals with Disabilities Act of 1988 was America's first-ever legislation specifically about technology and people with disabilities. It authorized modest sums of money for states to use in educating people with disabilities about products, and in putting technology experts in touch with individuals who need those devices. States receiving Tech Act money must obey Section 508 of the Rehabilitation Act. Section 508 requires that any office equipment or information services purchased, leased, rented, or otherwise acquired by federal agencies and by units of government in states receiving Tech Act monies must be accessible to and usable by individuals with disabilities.

If we decide to expand our national commitment to making technology more readily available to all Americans with disabilities, we will have to go well beyond the current policy as expressed in the Tech Act and in Section 508. Are we prepared to do that? For example, we must enforce accessibility of all electronic products or computer-based services sold or made in the United States for individuals with disabilities — as has been done with buses, train cars, and buildings. In the so-called Information Age, we should not treat electronic products any differently than we now do public transit vehicles and aspects of the built environment.

Marcia Scherer's contribution in this volume is to illuminate these issues for us by showing how they emerge in the real lives of individual human beings. As tantalizing as many of the emerging technologies are, we cannot just hand them to people with disabilities, any more than we can introduce Coca Cola bottles into a culture that has no organized disposal system. The introduction of high technology into the lives of individuals with disabilities often has unexpected and indeed unforeseeable consequences. That is why Dr. Scherer emphasizes that technology alone seldom is the answer.

Still, we are asking questions that never occurred to me when I was trying to accommodate Rita Varela's typing limitations. Marcia Scherer's gift to us in this book is that she stimulates us to ask good questions. As always, the hard part is not to answer but to ask the right questions.

Frank G. Bowe, Ph.D., LL.D. is a Dr. Mervin Livingston Schloss Distinguished Professor, at the Department of Counseling, Research, Special Education and Rehabilitation, School of Education and Allied Human Services, Hofstra University. His 1984 book Personal Computers and Special Needs *was the first text on high technology and persons with disabilities.*

Introduction

by Peter Axelson

People whose function is so limited that assistive technologies are essential for their functioning have the highest rate of assistive technology usage. For others whose technology use is more optional, psychological factors, including everything from their background to their acceptance of their loss of function, will affect the choices they make regarding assistive and adaptive equipment.

Marcia Scherer theorizes that individuals must acknowledge their loss of function before they are willing to seek out, use, or design assistive devices. People may reject an assistive device because it identifies them as having a disability. To be effective, Scherer emphasizes, assistive technology must not only foster independence and autonomy but also contribute to a positive identity and enhanced self-esteem.

Assistive technology experts are truly in a unique position to improve and change the lives of the people they work with. With these clients, they can serve as facilitators, enabling clients to use assistive devices to make their lives work better. "People with disabilities have found assistive technology to be important enablers in achieving a high quality of life."

Scherer suggests these ways to improve users' attitudes toward assistive technology:

1. Give users more information about the advantages and disadvantages of specific technologies;

2. Give people a trial period to use a new device in the environment — home, work, outdoors — where they will use the device in their lives;

3. Schedule follow-up visits to help consumers refine and tune a device for their specific needs;

4. Put new users in touch with peers who use similar technology;

5. When training new users of technology, end each training session with a positive experience."There has been an explosion of the number and types of assistive technology and an expansion of their flexibility," Scherer notes. She suggests that users should have a

greater role in the design and prototyping of technology if it is to be more functional and better accepted by those it is intended to serve. Above all, her book emphasizes, the technology, however helpful it may be in its design, cannot function without acceptance from potential users.

Peter Axelson, M.S.M.E., is Director of Research & Development, Beneficial Designs, Minden, Nevada.

Author's Introduction

*"There ain't nothin' worse than being stuck. There's nothin'
you can do to change it physically and you know that right off
the bat. And when you ain't got nothin' to fight with, then you
lose your will."*

— BUTCH, a 38-year-old man with paralysis from a spinal cord
   injury received in an automobile accident, speaking four
   years after his injury

For many individuals with disabilities, life itself depends on a pacemaker, a ventilator, or a kidney dialysis machine. Technology has enabled others to speak for the first time in their lives, to get around independently even though unable to walk, to read books any time and anywhere, and to communicate with anyone in the world even though they are without sight or hearing. Technology has helped people with physical disabilities more than they ever thought possible — not just to survive severe illness and trauma, but to function as if they had no physical limitation.

Technology has become smarter, smaller, lighter in weight, and many devices have become more affordable. Since the mid-1970s, the development of devices to enhance the independent functioning of individuals with disabilities has grown at a rapid rate. Called "assistive devices" or "assistive technologies," these devices have become a very important part of the education and rehabilitation of people with disabilities; so much so that each piece of federal legislation passed since 1988 regarding persons with disabilities mandates their consideration.

Assistive technologies include wheelchairs, magnifying and other reading devices, and equipment for eating and grooming. The list covers all areas of functioning and is extensive; whole catalogs and web sites exist which identify and describe the thousands of devices available. But as useful as these resources are in describing available technologies and how they work, there is comparatively little information on how the devices affect the individuals who use them. Nor is there much information available on how one matches individuals with disabilities with the most appropriate devices to enhance their independent functioning and goal achievement, or how to support technology adoption so fewer devices go unused or become discarded.

This book has been written to help address just such needs. It describes the lives of people who use assistive devices, as well as the lives of those who have tried them and abandoned their use. Rather than a technical description of the various devices available, this book is concerned with telling the stories of why people with disabilities use and don't use assistive devices, as well as the advantages and the limitations they perceive from their use. People who have abandoned devices, or chose not to try them, are a matter of great concern because they indicate that devices are not always seen as helpful by those for whom professionals deem them suitable. Why this is so is a major concern of this book.

Technology is meant to free people — to allow people to extend their abilities and manage their lives more efficiently and effectively. It has raised the hopes of many for a better and easier life. This is just as true for people with physical disabilities. However, the physical freedom offered by many technical advances has not resulted in the improved quality of life that many envisioned. This book shows how, paradoxically, the more technology became available and the freer from physical limitations individuals with disabilities became, the more *stuck* many seemed in several important ways.

The purpose of this book, then, is to give voices to the users of assistive technology, and thereby to educate their friends, their families, and the professionals who work with them. All of us need to understand better how to introduce and support the use of this technology to improve the *quality of life* of those with disabilities. While machines and assistive devices provide important assistance to persons with disabilities, individuals must be prepared and trained to use those devices that were designed to be useful for them. They should be counseled to help them understand their current situation, the vast array of opportunities and possibilities available to them, and the contribution technologies can offer. They require ongoing consultation so the proper use of devices can be monitored and adjusted as users' needs and preferences change. This counseling and consultation place the user at the *center* of the process of providing assistive technology to persons with disabilities.

The best use of technologies is achieved by matching devices to persons, not vice versa, and the use of a "person first" perspective. Doing otherwise invites the avoidance or abandonment of devices.

TECHNOLOGY IS THE ANSWER,
BUT THAT'S NOT THE QUESTION

It was 1977, the year I received my master's degree in rehabilitation counseling; my husband, an electrical engineer, was reading an article in a trade journal about computerized devices to help people with disabilities. "Here's an article I'd like you to read. I think this is going to be a big thing in the future," he said.

He certainly was right! I read that article, and all the others he passed on to me. Interestingly, it would be several years before articles on such assistive devices would appear in my rehabilitation journals. As time went on, I became increasingly concerned that issues of *quality of life* — individuals' emotional, personal, and social goals — were being neglected in favor of technical solutions to the needs and preferences consumers presented to their rehabilitation agencies. I made the decision to try and find out more.

It was for the purpose of pursuing research in such quality of life issues that the National Science Foundation awarded me a grant to study the perspectives and experiences of people with disabilities living with assistive devices, and the impact of the devices on their quality of life. I worked with a small group of people with disabilities. At the time of my initial study in 1986, all were adults between the ages of 21 and 45, half of who were born with their disability (cerebral palsy); the remainder had acquired their disability in adulthood (spinal cord injury). In addition to interviewing and observing them, I also spoke with their rehabilitation engineers and primary therapists.

Brief description of the original study[1]

Participants were observed in their rehabilitation centers, homes, or work sites to understand how they performed with or without the use of assistive technologies in their daily activities. Observation and interview notes were kept on whether or not they used assistive technologies; on the ease, comfort and effectiveness of use; and on the conditions and circumstances under which they experienced difficulties. Additionally, each respondent completed a number of measures:

Assessment of Physical Functioning — The Personal Capacities Questionnaire (PCQ) developed by the University of Minnesota's Rehabilitation Research and Training Center is a 30-item global functional assessment inventory covering communication, motor, physical, adaptive behavior, and vocational factors (Crewe & Dijkers, 1995). Ratings reflect current functioning with or without the use of AT.

Assessment of Personal Characteristics — The Taylor-Johnson Temperament Analysis (TJTA) is a 180-item instrument that provides a personality profile of an individual on the following nine scales: Nervous, depressive, active-social, expressive-responsive, sympathetic, subjective, dominant, hostile and self-disciplined. It also assesses six trait patterns: Anxiety, withdrawal, hostile-dominant, dependent-hostile, emotionally inhibited/emotionally repressed, and a socially effective pattern. The TJTA was chosen because it assumes a normal personality, not psychopathology.

The Defense Mechanism Inventory (DMI) is an objective paper-and-pencil inventory to measure the degrees to which participants "passively" cope with (internalize, repress) and "actively" cope with (externalize, express) frustration.

Assessment of Social Support — The Inventory of Socially Supportive Behaviors (ISSB) is a 40-item questionnaire assessing the frequency of social support experienced during the preceding four-week period (e.g., Novack and Gage, 1995).

The individuals who participated in the original study, who have met and talked with me for over 18 years, are truly transition people. For the most part they grew up during the pre-mainstreaming and pre-inclusion years before people with disabilities were extended civil rights. Many of them are pioneers in the use of assistive devices and worked actively with their therapists — and continue to do so — to fabricate or customize their own equipment. To keep these persons more clearly in mind as they emerge in the narrative, I have summarized key information about them in a chart at the end of Chapter Two. The reader who wishes to follow the story of a particular individual will find page references under that person's name in the Index.

This book portrays these persons for almost two decades from the 20th century into the 21st century; a time span that is special because it encompasses a period of great cultural, social, political and economic changes impacting the lives of each of us. Many of the issues and problems recounted in this book didn't exist before the 1980s; some may now be resolved or nonexistent while others have worsened. For now, they define the lives of almost all people with physical disabilities. By the time these accounts are read, the individuals in this book will have likely changed again, as they formulate new perspectives and experiences in an ongoing developmental process and in an ever-changing context.

The majority of assistive technologies are used for mobility: according to the 1994 U.S. National Health Interview Survey approximately 7.4 million people in the U.S. use some type of mobility technology. Individuals with spinal cord injuries or with cerebral palsy are examples of persons for whom mobility devices are appropriate. People with cerebral palsy may also use communication devices. Individuals in both groups use a variety of devices for personal care, writing, recreation, and so on.

In the first two chapters, the functional, personal, and psychosocial aspects of the lives of persons who received their spinal cord injuries in adulthood (Chapter One) are compared to those of persons born with cerebral palsy (Chapter Two). Chapter Three describes the representative types of assistive technologies available today — some of the more than 20,000 different devices on the market.

Policies, attitudes, and opportunities do not develop in a vacuum. They evolve over time in a social, political and economic milieu. Chapter Four traces the history of the care and rehabilitation given to individuals with disabilities in the United States. While governmental policies and social attitudes have oscillated over time in their degree of humanitarianism, we are currently at a point, thanks in part to assistive devices, when people with disabilities are becoming more visible throughout society. Visibility, however, is one thing; inclusion and participation are quite another.

Chapter Five presents differing perspectives of rehabilitation success and presents arguments as to why the definitions of *"rehabilitation success"* need to be changed: not just society's definition, but also the definitions used by rehabilitation professionals and by people with disabilities themselves.

Chapter Six discusses the concept of *quality of life* and illustrates the concept with examples from the lives of several individuals with disabilities. While their issues and concerns are individualized, they share concerns around independence and interdependence.

Chapter Seven discusses the ways in which people learn to live with their disabilities. Individuals respond in ways that reflect learned patterns for satisfying their needs, their personal characteristics, and the expectations others have of them. Some may experience cycles of hope; others despair; most, periods of both hope and despair. These influence one's view of opportunities, growth, and the use of technological and other assistance. Taken as a whole, they eventually characterize a person's quality of life.

In Chapter Eight, the reasons people with disabilities give for using or not using assistive devices are discussed. Approximately one-third of assistive technologies are discarded by their users. Sometimes this is because the person no longer needs it, but far too often a technology is abandoned because it doesn't meet a person's expectations, needs, or preferences. This section focuses on recommendations to improve this situation and to enhance the overall quality of life of persons with disabilities.

Chapter Nine first brings us current on the individuals in the book. We see the changes in their lives and their frustrations as they confront challenges with their health, family, and the services they must depend on. Beyond that, they discuss their needs for belonging, for intimacy with other persons, and their sense of being stuck in their situations — without feeling they can break out into a more enhanced quality of life.

Finally, Chapter Ten addresses the more general issues confronting all persons with disabilities as we have entered the 21st century.

Throughout this book, I present the experiences, ideas, and hopes of people with disabilities, as well as their therapists and engineers, in their own words,[2] so as to help give their voices a forum. Though the names and other identifying features of the persons quoted throughout this book have been changed to protect their privacy, their statements and experiences have not been altered in any way.

— Marcia J. Scherer
September 2004

Footnotes: Author's Introduction

1 The details of the study, the measures used, and its results are presented in Scherer (1988a, 1988b, 1990).

2 Terms used in 1986, when some of the original research was conducted, have been updated to reflect current preferences in terminology. I have tried to select words that are familiar to most readers, yet which put persons first and are not stigmatizing.

Footnotes in this edition can be found at the end of each chapter.

Acknowledgments

I owe much gratitude to the individuals who participated in my research project (whose names have been changed in this book to protect their privacy). In addition to them, I thank the following:

- The National Science Foundation for sponsoring the original study upon which this book is based

- Faculty at the University of Rochester and the National Technical Institute for the Deaf for their helpful guidance — especially Drs. Thomas Knapp (now at Ohio State) and Barbara McKee

- Dr. Milton Budoff, Publisher, Brookline Books, for his patience and invaluable guidance — and for publishing a line of books which share the purpose of advocating for persons with disabilities

- Jan Rowe, MPH, OTR/L, Associate Professor in the Department of Occupational Therapy at the University of Alabama at Birmingham School of Health Related Professions, for providing updated statistics on spinal cord injury and for writing the section on *Sexuality and SCI*

- Colleagues, students and consumers who over the years have shared their insights, comments and experiences

- And, finally, my deepest appreciation — as well as affection — to John Scherer, who truly started it all

The material in this book is based upon work supported in 1985-1986 by the National Science Foundation under grant RII-8512418 sponsored by the Ethics and Values in Science and Technology, and Biotechnology and Research to Aid the Handicapped programs. Additional material has been added to this book thanks to grant support from the American Association of Spinal Cord Injury Psychologists and Social Workers; National Institutes of Health, National Institute of Child Health and Human Development, National Center for Medical Rehabilitation Research; and National Institute for Disability and Rehabilitation Research. Funding from these sources has enabled me to continue my focus on ways to make *assistive technology* better suit and serve its users.
— M.J.S.

CHAPTER ONE

Going Into the 21st Century with a Disability

What man that sees the ever-whirling wheel
Of Change, the which all mortal things doth sway,
But that thereby doth find, and plainly feel,
How Mutability in them doth play
Her cruel sports, to many men's decay?
— EDMUND SPENSER

Imagine that you are suddenly unable to perform your usual activities, to go out to dinner with friends, to laugh and talk about something that happened at work, to cut your own steak and feed yourself. Then imagine having *never* done these things, even though you're 20 years old.

This is reality today for millions of Americans. And tomorrow it will be reality for more — perhaps someone very close to you.

This book shows — through the experiences of many persons who "tell it like it is" — what life is like today for individuals with severe physical disabilities such as spinal cord injuries and cerebral palsy. For example, 29-year-old Chuck was having an average day until, in the span of just a few hours, he left a rather carefree life of riding his motorcycle, tending bar, and hanging out with friends for one where he will never again be able to walk, feed himself, even go to the bathroom alone. Four years after his accident, Chuck's story, in his own words, tells what his life is like and how it is very different from anything he had ever imagined — totally unable to move or control a single muscle between the tops of his shoulders and the tips of his toes.

CHUCK, 1986

Before... okay, I was only tending bar. But to me, I was a success. I was happy with my life at the time. I didn't plan on being a bartender forever, but for then it was just the right thing I needed to get away from the stress of business. And I was having a good time. Probably the best time of my life.

I'd been separated from my wife for a year and a half. Late one night, I was riding my motorcycle, and the next thing I knew I was in the hospital. I never knew what happened, and no one else was ever able to figure it out. My best guess is that some guy ran me off the road and I crashed.

I was aware of being sandwiched between two slices of board and being turned every couple of hours. My spleen and one kidney were gone. I could speak and hear and see, but that was about it. The thing was, I didn't even know what was going on. I was still confused about myself and my condition and I had everyone coming in and saying, "We're going to educate you to do this, help you to do that." I didn't even know what I wanted to do, could do, at that point.

For someone like me, paralyzed from the shoulders down, therapy should have been more practical — like taking us out to a grocery store or something like that where there are people around. And I wish I'd had counseling regularly... on a fairly regular basis. I'm not sure what would've come out of it, but if you see someone enough, eventually you're going to say something — try to bring things out, some of the anger, and things like that. That was something that was never done, and that anger just sits in there and grows.

Oh, they did have a psychologist on the floor. I think his name was Lloyd. I saw him once, and the major reason for that was because I smoke and didn't want to quit. He came in and said, "Well, maybe we should mark down whenever you have a cigarette." For Christ's sake. Didn't he see that I couldn't smoke without someone on the floor giving me one and holding it in my mouth for me?

From the moment of that accident on, I was no longer an independent person. It's like... I have a typewriter, to use an example. Okay, now I know that everyday I should spend some time putting the mouthstick in and just keep pounding on it — even if it's just 25 minutes — to keep the endurance in my neck up. But I don't always do that. Twenty-five minutes just goes somewhere else. I'll say, "I think I'll go have an extra cup of coffee." Other times I'll get involved and work for two hours straight. It's no different from when I was out in the business world working. I mean there were things I probably should've done, and I'd say, "I think I'll go have an extra cup of coffee," or "I'll do it tomorrow." And everybody does the same thing. But when you're in this condition, people say to you, "You've got to do it NOW." They don't look at it like they're looking at themselves, and saying, "I can put it off until later." No, it's "Let's do it now" with "You have to do this, you have to maintain that." Screw it! I'll do it when I get to it. I wasn't that organized before, so why should it change now? I know what has to be done and when it has to be done and that's what I work on. Your basic style doesn't change just because you're in a wheelchair and the only things you can move are from the neck up.

I was in a state of shock all through rehab, and truthfully, I'm still in a state of shock. Sometimes I sit here and ask, "Why did I ever live through this?" I think I'm depressed a little bit more... more than 50% of the time.

To get myself out of it, I make myself do something to get away from the four walls that are closing in. So, there's the TV again. Do you know what I mean? Before the accident, I never watched that much TV, and after, it's like, "There it is again."

I've talked with lots of quads, about my level, and everyone seems to agree they would rather have not been saved than to be in the situation they're in now... to be so dependent. And there are a lot of times I feel the same way.

I try to make the best of what I've got, but on the other hand, I look at my friends that I used to play football with, or baseball, or something, and they're still doing it. I go out to lunch with them now and get treated like a helpless kid or something. And that makes me feel even worse. Because then I wish that I could stand up, just for a couple of minutes, so I could tell them to shove off.

But when you're in this condition, you have to accept their ideas of help to a certain extent so your friends don't feel too guilty. You have to let them accept it on their own level. At least that's my experience, with my friends.

On the romantic side, women have a tendency to move away from me... It's like, "See ya later." I mean, it's easy to find someone to say, "Okay, let's go out," but when it comes to the romantic side of it, they're not sure what to do or what to expect. It's hard to approach somebody when you're in a wheelchair, as opposed to the way it was before. I mean, what do you say? Can I buy you a drink, and by the way, would you help me with mine?

Even my one-year-old niece. She doesn't understand the wheelchair and so she's kinda leery of it. And I just wish she'd come up and grab me and give me a hug.

I find now that I identify with people with disabilities a little bit more than I did before. Even after my open heart surgery and car accident, I was always the type of person, if I saw someone in a wheelchair, I was probably like anyone else and it was like, "Hi, how're you doing." I wasn't really careful with what I was saying. I did know a couple of guys in wheelchairs and I look at them a lot different now than before. Then, I'd kid around a little and things like that and now it's more like I really know what they're talking about when they say things.

I seem to notice people a lot more, too. Even someone on crutches sticks out more to me now than in the past. It's not like I look over their heads anymore and just cruise on by. Now I search their faces... and look more in their eyes.

Chuck's experience highlights not only many of the physical and functional issues a person with a spinal cord injury must confront, but also the often unexamined emotional and social issues encountered by a person with disabilities.

The latter two issues will be a chief focus of this book, but before going into these issues in detail, I want to briefly review what is currently known about spinal cord injuries and the range of limitations in function they can cause.

SPINAL CORD INJURIES: DEMOGRAPHICS, PHYSICAL EFFECTS, AND FUNCTIONAL EXPECTATIONS

Chuck is just one of approximately 49.5 million Americans with disabilities according to the U.S. Census Bureau (2000). The National Council on Disability clarifies that this number is not inclusive of children birth to 5 years of age, which could be several million more people (M. Gould, personal communication, June 16, 2004). In addition to disabilities arising from genetics, disease, and the aging process, hazards of modern living (vehicle accidents, falls, and other traumas) cause severe injuries that people are surviving, but with permanent disabilities. Survival rates have been enhanced by improvements in vehicle occupant protection, developments in emergency medical care and very early intervention by emergency medical personnel, specialized trauma centers, and multidisciplinary rehabilitation centers. Advances in the control of infections and other conditions secondary to a traumatic spinal cord injury have also served to increase the likelihood that persons with severe spinal cord injuries can live well beyond middle-age.

The generally accepted data in 2004 regarding the incidence (number of new spinal cord injuries each year) is 11,000 injuries. The prevalence of spinal cord injuries (total number of individuals living with SCI in a population during a given year) is between 219,000 and 279,000 persons in the US. (National Spinal Cord Injury Statistical Center, Centers for Disease Control and Prevention, 2003). Tetraplegics (those, like Chuck, who are paralyzed from the shoulders down) comprise just over half of these individuals living with spinal cord injuries.

As Chuck said when talking about his hospital stay, "... everyone was coming in and saying, 'We're going to educate you to do this, help you to do that.'" In comprehensive rehabilitation units, available throughout the U.S., each spinal-cord-injured patient has an entire team of professionals working to help preserve and enhance as much sensation and as many motor and other functional capabilities as possible. This team may consist of physicians specializing in emergency, internal, neurological, orthopedic, urological, and rehabilitation medicine; it may also include nurses, physical therapists, occupational therapists, social workers, psychologists, and vocational rehabilitation counselors. If the individual is fortunate enough to be in a specialized spinal cord injury center, the individual has this team from the very beginning. The usual course of treatment begins with stabilization of the person's medical condition and the treatment of associated injuries. Then the person is taught ways to be physically independent in spite of what may be serious functional limitations, as well as how to perform self-care activities, avoid infection and prevent additional health problems. Finally, the team guides the individual through discharge planning and assists in planning follow-up care once the person is back in the community.

The many causes of spinal cord injuries basically fall into two broad categories: pathological (due to disease processes) and traumatic (due to injury). Such pathologies as transverse myelitis, infection (abscess), and tumors can permanently damage the spinal cord, which is the main pathway for the nerves to the neck, arms, diaphragm, thorax, abdomen, pelvis, and legs. Traumatic spinal cord injuries originate from automobile and motorcycle accidents, sports injuries, gunshot wounds, and falls, with the greatest increase seen in injuries as a result of violence.

Over time, the proportions of individuals served by specialized spinal cord injury centers may differ in these two categories as well as by the type of pathology or trauma. In 1984, for example, in the category of traumatic spinal cord injuries, Rochester, NY, had mostly injuries from automobile accidents. During the same year, sports injuries predominated on the West Coast (Scherer, 1984). Mandated safety and protective measures have led to decreasing numbers of injuries from automobile crashes and sports injuries, yet motor vehicle crashes have remained the most common cause of spinal cord injury. In a presentation of statistics collected in the U.S. from 1973 to 2003, DeVivo, Jackson, Dijkers and Poczatek (2004) showed that there has been an increase in the *percentage* of injuries due to falls, from 16.5% prior to 1980 to 23.8% since 2000. While sports injuries in general have declined over time, there has been an increase in the number of injuries due to snow skiing. Injuries from bicycle, ATV, and motorcycle accidents have also increased. In 2000, the number of spinal cord injuries resulting from violence, almost all from gunshot wounds, started to trend downward to only 11.2% of all causes of SCI.

Due to the nature of the primary causes of traumatic spinal cord injuries, statistics show that men are involved at a rate four times that of women. Other data from the Spinal Cord Injury Information Network (2000) indicate that 53% of SCIs occur among persons in the 16 to 30 year age group, and the average age at injury is 32.6 years. Since 1973 there has been an increase in the mean age at time of injury (from 28.6 prior to 1979 to 32.6 today). Another trend is an increase in the proportion of those who were at least 61 years of age at injury. In the 1970s persons older than 60 years of age at injury comprised 4.7% of the database. Since 2000 this has increased to 11.4%. This is consistent with the rising number of injuries due to falls. Among those injured since 2000, 59.1% were Caucasian, 27.6% were African-American, 7.7% were Hispanics, 0.4% were American Indian, 2.1% were Asian, and 0.5% were unknown (Spinal Cord Injury Statistical Center, Centers for Disease Control and Prevention, 2003).

The course of each spinal cord injury is unique: Similar injuries often do not result in the same losses of motor function and sensation. Also, individuals react and adjust to their injuries in a variety of ways and over varying lengths of time (Krause & Crewe, 1987; Trieschmann, 1988). Several factors are used to define and classify types of spinal cord injuries anatomically and functionally. They also serve as a guide for planning treatment. The International Standards for Neurological and Functional Classification of Spinal Cord Injury (ASIA, 1996) is generally accepted as the preferred system for evaluating and classifying SCI. It indicates both the location of the injury along the spinal cord and the lowest muscle with normal function. For the purpose of this classification by functional level, the spinal cord has been sectioned into four zones: from top to bottom, *cervical, thoracic, lumbar, and sacral.*

As shown in Figure 1-1, there are many segments within each zone. For example, the cervical (C) zone has eight segments that serve the neck, arm and diaphragm. The highest injury within the cervical zone (and along the entire spinal cord, since the cervical zone is the highest zone) is in the upper neck area and is classified C1; the lowest (in the upper back area) is C8. The C7 vertebra can be felt easily at the base of the neck; it protrudes further than any other.

"Incomplete" injuries suggest that some sensation (the capability to receive information from or through the body) and/or some controlled motor function (the capability to make one's muscles and body act) has been preserved or has returned below the zone of injury. A person with an incomplete injury may be able to feel heat or someone's touch, and may only have numbness or weakness in affected muscles instead of paralysis. If there is preserved sensation only, then the person has some sensation below the level of injury, but complete loss of voluntary motor control. "Complete" injuries indicate that the spinal cord has been so severely cut, bruised or crushed that there has been no preservation of either motor function or sensation below the zone of injury. Involuntary muscle control — the kind that keeps our hearts beating without us

Figure 1-1: Spinal Cord Injury Functional Outcomes Chart

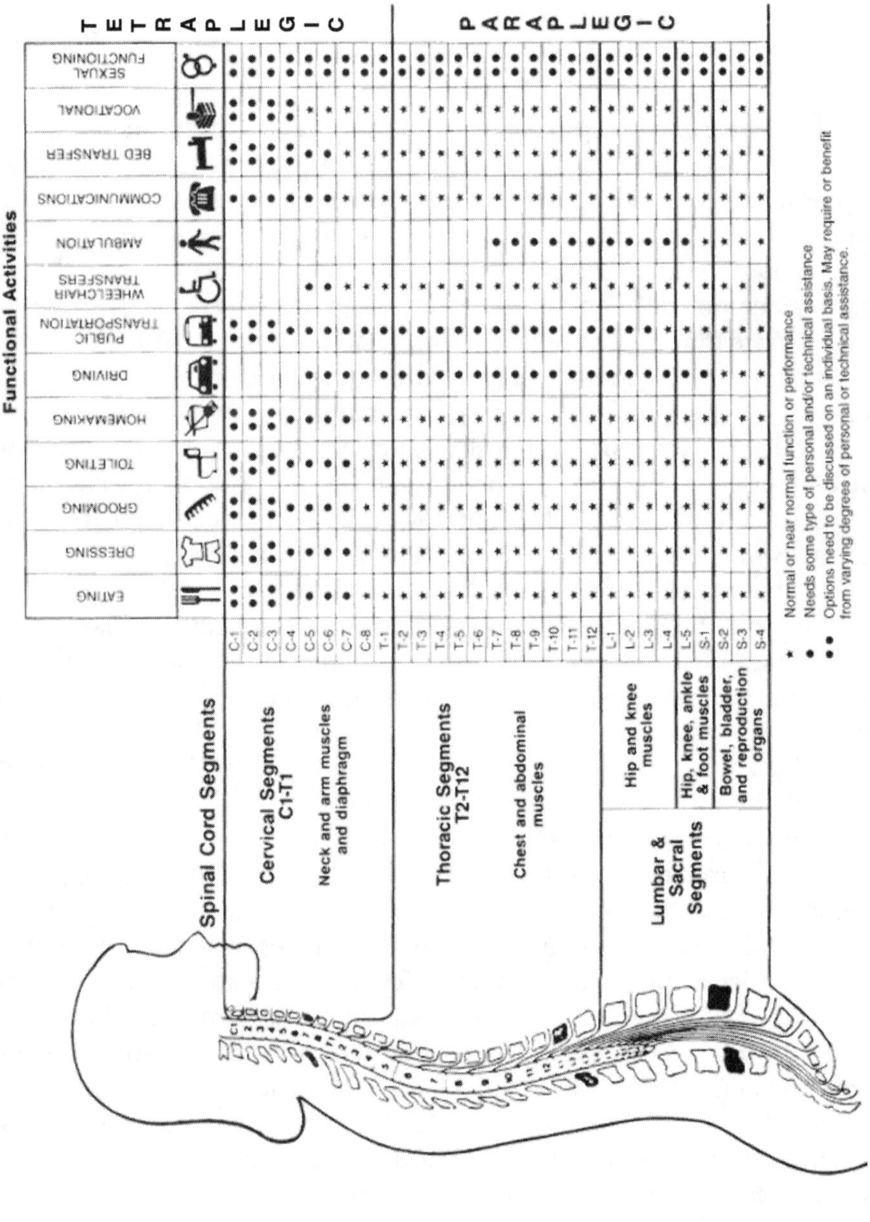

Functional Activities

TETRAPLEGIC PARAPLEGIC

Functional Activities (rows, listed):
SEXUAL FUNCTIONING
VOCATIONAL
BED TRANSFER
COMMUNICATIONS
AMBULATION
WHEELCHAIR TRANSFERS
PUBLIC TRANSPORTATION
DRIVING
HOMEMAKING
TOILETING
GROOMING
DRESSING
EATING

Spinal cord segment columns:
C-1, C-2, C-3, C-4, C-5, C-6, C-7, C-8, T-1, T-2, T-3, T-4, T-5, T-6, T-7, T-8, T-9, T-10, T-11, T-12, L-1, L-2, L-3, L-4, L-5, S-1, S-2, S-3, S-4

Spinal Cord Segments

Cervical Segments C1-T1 — Neck and arm muscles and diaphragm

Thoracic Segments T2-T12 — Chest and abdominal muscles

Lumbar & Sacral Segments:
- Hip and knee muscles
- Hip, knee, ankle & foot muscles
- Bowel, bladder, and reproduction organs

Legend:
* Normal or near normal function or performance
•• Needs some type of personal and/or technical assistance
••• Options need to be discussed on an individual basis. May require or benefit from varying degrees of personal or technical assistance.

having to think about it — is a brain activity and, thus, is not paralyzed by a spinal cord injury. Advances in trauma and medical care have resulted in increasing numbers of incomplete rather than complete injuries. People have a greater chance of recovering motor and sensory function if they have an incomplete lesion at the time of injury (Rehabilitation Research and Training Center on Secondary Conditions of SCI and Model SCI Care Center, 2000).

Figure 1-1 presents expectations of the functional outcomes of people with motor complete SCI at 1 year after injury (Consortium for Spinal Cord Medicine, 1999). Chuck has a C4 complete injury and is paralyzed from the shoulders down, with little or no sensation or motor function anywhere below the level of his injury; as shown in the chart, he requires a good deal of assistance for most functional activities. Persons with injuries at the C5 and C6 levels fare better (Yarkony & Chen, 1996). They can be expected to perform some activities like eating and propelling a manual wheelchair independently and can drive a van with a lift, modified controls and other adapted equipment. Individuals with an injury at the C7 or C8 level may work with their hands independently, and they have functioning triceps (the upper, outer arm muscles we feel when doing push-ups) to get themselves in and out of their wheelchairs independently. The presence or absence of functional triceps is a critical determinant for functional independence in self-care tasks (Welch, Lobley, O'Sullivan & Freed, 1986).

Cervical spinal cord injuries result in a condition known as *tetraplegia*. (The older term, "quadriplegia," is now less preferred as a description of muscular paralysis in all four quadrants of the body — both arms, both legs.) *Paraplegia* refers to paralysis in the body's two lower quadrants — indicating that the person has little voluntary movement below the waist and has paralysis in both legs. Spinal cord injuries at the mid-thoracic level or below frequently result in paraplegia.The lower the functional level of the injury, the more voluntary motor control and muscle power are available to the individual. Trends over time indicate an increasing proportion of persons with incomplete paraplegia and a decreasing proportion of persons with complete tetraplegia. This is due, no doubt, to advances in vehicle occupant protection and in emergency medicine.

Hemiplegia is a term that also indicates paralysis, but on one side of the body or the other. "Right-sided hemiplegia" means a person has paralysis of the right side, including the right arm and leg. Hemiplegia is *not* an outcome of a spinal cord injury; it is the result of an injury to the side of the brain opposite the side of weakness or paralysis — i.e., right-sided paralysis indicates the brain was injured in the left hemisphere. Strokes, tumors, birth injuries (such as cerebral palsy), and other traumatic injuries to the brain may cause damage that can lead to hemiplegia or, if more severe, to tetraplegia.

Uncontrolled movements, such as simple reflexes, can cause a person's legs to move or jerk in response to stimulation — sometimes nothing more than the touch of bed clothing. This is called *spastic paralysis*. It can make the leg, for example, quiver and jerk uncontrollably for several minutes at a time. Unfortunately, such spasticity is not an indication that motor functioning is returning. Rather than being a positive sign, these spasms or uncontrollable episodes of jerking are more a source of annoyance and embarrassment to individuals who may have such spastic reactions many times a day. For this reason, many individuals with spastic paralysis are given muscle relaxants, such as Valium or baclofen, to reduce the frequency and duration of spastic episodes.

When Chuck was in rehabilitation for his spinal cord injury in 1982, the average length of stay was over 100 days. Now it is under 44 days in most cases. After their discharge, 88-90% of all persons with SCI return home and less than 5% are discharged to nursing homes. The remaining are discharged to hospitals, group living situations or other destinations (Rehabilitation Research and Training Center on Secondary Conditions of SCI and Model SCI Care Center, 2000). This high rate of discharge to home has been made possible to a great extent by the availability of assistance from caretakers and technologies. Data from the 1990 National Health Interview Survey on Assistive Devices (NHIS-AD) showed that in that year more than 13 million Americans with disabilities (about 5.3% of the population) used assistive devices. By group, the majority of devices used were for mobility (6.4 million), with 1.4 million persons using wheelchairs (LaPlante, Hendershot, & Moss, 1992).

A Spinal Cord Injury is a Lifelong Health Condition

Even such explicit terms as *tetraplegia* and C4 *complete* can be applied to a variety of patterns of functioning. One such pattern is represented by Chuck, whose spinal cord is damaged at the C4 level, and who has voluntary control only of the muscles of his neck, face, and head. Chuck fits the C4 profile in Figure 1-1 perfectly. Unlike some C4-injured individuals, Chuck can breathe without the assistance of a ventilator. Besides having little controllable movement, Chuck has no sensation of any type below his level of injury, including the ability to feel pain, temperature changes, and touch. Thus, Chuck can no longer shave or dress himself. He requires help from assistive devices and from others — either family members, friends, or hired personal assistants — for all of his eating, bathing, dressing, and grooming needs. Getting around requires the use of a wheelchair.

From Chuck's standpoint, his environment is "totally controlled." His privacy is essentially nonexistent. When he wants a cigarette, he needs someone to light it, hold it to his lips, and extinguish it. Because of his inability to move at will and his lack of sensation, he has no control over his bladder and bowel. A spinal cord injury — for Chuck and for all people with severe high level spinal cord injuries — is a lifelong health condition that requires regular and serious attention to prescribed daily programs of diet control, rest, physical exercise, and personal hygiene. Otherwise, such preventable and treatable conditions as pressure sores, respiratory problems, coronary disease, urinary tract and kidney infections are apt to create serious and recurring medical problems that can lead to frequent hospitalization, chronic periods of interrupted time from work or a training program, and even premature death (Yarkony & Chen, 1996).

The Hospital Often Becomes a Second Home

When Chuck and I first met, it was four years after his accident, but he was in the hospital again for several months recovering from a surgical procedure. While we were talking, hospital professionals of many types came in to chat and kid with him and inquire into his physical needs — and, I remember thinking, to be protective of him. Once my tape recorder had been spotted, my ID badge was scrutinized by one of Chuck's young, freshly trained attending physicians who, in a very polite yet firm professional manner, inquired into my identity and purpose for being in Chuck's room. Clearly, they cared about Chuck's well-being and were guarding against his being made uncomfortable or being exploited in any way.

At one point during another of our conversations, a nurse came in with some medication, dispensed with the following plea: "No more tricks now, okay."

I was curious to know what she was referring to, so I asked Chuck what she had meant. "You aren't one of those guys that uses the cheek as a pouch and then spits out the pills later, are you?" I was aware, even as I asked the question, that it sounded flip, insensitive.

No. She was talking about the night I had the Code Blues. I went into cardiac arrest. They think it was a reaction to one of the medications they gave me. But they don't really know for sure what happened. I wish they did.

Chuck's matter-of-fact tone and acceptance of this emergency situation startled me. Perhaps he sensed this.

> Oh, that wasn't the first time that's happened. A couple of other times I've died and been resuscitated.

Chuck, just 33 years old, was certainly no stranger to hospitals — nor apparently to physical distress and even death. At age 19 he had open heart surgery for a blocked aorta. Eight months after his heart surgery, he was in an automobile accident and sustained lower back injuries. He was 29 years old when he had the motorcycle accident that resulted in his C4 spinal cord injury, and he has been in and out of the hospital since. In addition to his heart problems, he has lost his spleen and one kidney.

The calm, good-natured man in this room had certainly been through plenty of trials. Can it be surprising, then, that the hospital staff wanted to befriend him — and to protect and shield him from any further misfortune?

BRIAN, 1986

Today, a person with a spinal cord injury, especially an individual with voluntary movement in the arms and shoulders (injuries at the C6 level and below), can live and function with considerable independence. One example is Brian, who sustained an incomplete C6 spinal cord injury in a 1978 motorcycle accident, when he was 17 years old.

> It was a sunny, t-shirt and light jacket kind of day. I had finished a busy week moving people out of their apartments and into new ones, cutting people's lawns, painting houses and doing various odd jobs. I was 17, working as a rent-a-kid, and had a fast and busy schedule. The money was good that summer, but being a normal kid, I looked forward to the weekends.
>
> I had a few hours to kill and it was hard to stay inside on such a nice day. Sitting in the garage was a red and black Honda dirt bike which I had shared with my dad for the last two years. For Dad, it was simply a toy; for me, it was the one vehicle that gave me an adult-like freedom and independence. With a swift, even motion of my right foot on the kick start, I fired up the engine and headed out towards a well-known bike trail.
>
> Gunning the bike, I fishtailed from the trail onto a long-disused railroad bed; the tracks had been ripped out ten years earlier. I had an exhilarating sense of well-being as I headed west doing 35 m.p.h. in 3rd gear. That was the last thing I remember.
>
> After waking up from a two-week-long coma, the first thing I remember was lying face down on a Stryker Frame with 35 pounds of traction

bolted to my head and being rotated every so often. It was cold and bright. Saliva was dripping out of my mouth into a basin on the floor, and a respirator was attached to my throat pumping air into my lungs. My friends sat on the floor trying to keep me comfortable by just being there. I wasn't able to talk with all the drugs they put me on, plus my vocal cords were paralyzed. I didn't know where I was or what had happened at this point.

The days passed by in a continuous struggle to survive. I suffered three respiratory arrests, and at one time my heart stopped for 6 seconds.

I felt helpless in a body that wouldn't move. The doctors said there was little hope I would ever regain anything back. I had lost my memory and was like a child again. My mother would read to me every day. She read from the book *The Other Side of the Mountain*, which was a comfort and inspiration to me and to my mother. One day a few of my closest friends brought a cassette tape that included some of the music we always used to listen to, hoping it would engage some recognition of the past. Right before they would leave it would be turned on. All alone I would listen to Marshall Tucker, the Flying Burrito Brothers, and the Grateful Dead. After listening to the tape several times, small fragments of the past were piecing together.

Each day had its ups and downs, and slowly I was regaining my strength but, more importantly, my mind. For a while, I would communicate by use of a wordboard.

Four months had passed and I finally found myself on a rehabilitation floor. By that time my mind was in full flight, but still I was too weak to sit in a wheelchair. The first things I thought about were skiing, taking drives, and going to concerts, because those are the things I did with my friends. It wasn't a matter of 'How am I going to put on my pants again?' — things like that were really secondary.

My friends came up to visit as usual and said that my favorite group, the Grateful Dead, were playing here in November. My mind was back, but I had to get my strength. The doctors said I would have to sit 4 to 5 hours straight if I were to go to the concert. My ambition to go was strong and I had to work for it. Every time I got in the wheelchair, I blacked right out. Each day for only a short time I would sit in a semi-reclined position, determined to reach my goal. After a couple of days I was up to three hours. The day of the show I reached my goal and I was psyched. The concert was the first time I had been out of the hospital. I had reached my destination.

Thus began my second life. The first was one of standing and being active, and the second life is one of being in a wheelchair. The second life is the one where I realized you can't take life for granted. You have to make each day count to its fullest. That's why I try to accomplish at least a couple of things each day, even if they're small things.

At the time of this interview, Brian was single and living with his parents in his own apartment on one side of the family house. His father, an architect, constructed it especially for him, according to his own specifications. There is a private entryway into his two-room apartment — a bath and a bedroom/office — with a ramp leading from his door to the driveway.

> There's no other place around here that can match it, and a lot of the apartment buildings aren't accessible to people in chairs. Strangely enough, before my accident, I pictured having a room here. Everything was the same — the wood paneling, deerskin on the wall, stuffed owl, and the potbelly stove — except there were mountains in the back.

Looking around, I noticed that Brian's apartment overlooks a large wooded backyard with several bird feeders dangling from the branches of the trees nearest the house. Inside, he has a parakeet, several plants, and a sophisticated stereo system all in a space about the size of a large bedroom. In addition to the deerskin, his walls are covered with colorful posters, and the bright colors and variety of textures and shapes made his room look just like a student's dorm room as well as a mountain lodge.

His place was designed to be a serious work and study area, not a retreat, and his desk is crammed with several inches of books and papers strewn along the top. Brian is studying for a degree in manufacturing engineering technology and is, apparently, a good student: His employer for his cooperative work experience told Brian that he could expect a permanent job there upon the completion of his degree program.

Brian, while not what anyone would call a "handsome" man, is what everyone would consider an "attractive" man. He is very thin, almost gaunt. The preppie attire on such a lanky frame, combined with a well-trimmed beard, call forth images of sportsman-cum-student. He has no other medical conditions, and he takes "only typical quad medications like Valium for spasticity."

An average day for Brian starts when he pulls himself out of bed and into his power wheelchair with the assistance of an overhead trapeze bar. While he can move only his head, neck, shoulders and arms, he is able to groom and dress himself with the use of such aids as zipper pulls and Velcro closures on shirts and pants — and even his shoes, which he can grasp and slide onto his feet with a pistol-grip reacher. Once dressed, Brian goes into the kitchen to prepare and eat his breakfast. He then grabs a jacket and his books and heads out to his van — a vehicle designed to accommodate both him and his power wheelchair — which he operates by hand controls.

In the same way one opens the trunk of a car, Brian inserts a key (with a built-up handle) into a slot towards the rear of the passenger side of the van, activating a switch that slides open the side doors. Another turn of the key lowers a hydraulic lift. Brian removes the key, eases himself into place on the lift, and locks his wheelchair in place. He activates a switch to raise himself to the level of the floor of the van; once there, he activates another switch that automatically closes the door. Then he wheels into position behind the steering wheel, locks his wheelchair into place and, through adapted hand controls, starts the ignition and drives off to school and work. For Brian, this van is a major bridge to independence.

> I can't tell you how much my van has helped me see the light in so many ways. Before, I had the motorcycle — and I drove that every day. I had that independence, and all of a sudden it got struck down. Here I was stuck. I'm fortunate I had that [power wheelchair] to get me out when I needed to get out. Now that's just expanded with the van. I can come and go whenever I want to.

Once Brian arrives at school or work, he is able — thanks to ramps and elevators — to access almost any building, floor, and office he wishes. Once in his own office, a special desk allows his wheelchair to slide under it so that his wheelchair becomes his desk chair as well. On the desk is Brian's computer, which can give him access to anyone in just about any place in the world.

> It's mind-boggling when you think of the things that they're coming up with. What higher-level quads like me couldn't do before, we can do now. What a big incentive to keep going. There are so many advantages.... I mean, I'm glad I broke my neck in this century!"

Brian places a high value on his assistive devices and sees them as keys to his independence. When I told him that some people choose not to use them, he seemed surprised.

> Eventually, what people see as optional devices now are going to be seen as essential. I'm shocked to hear that some people would actually turn something down that's available to upgrade their functioning. And I'm curious why. It totally baffles me.

In spite of Brian's many assistive devices and his independence, he acknowledges that a lot of physical and emotional challenges remain.

It takes twice as long, three times as long for me to do a simple thing [like getting in his van and driving off to work]. It takes a lot of time and definitely a lot of patience, especially when things aren't going right. There are times when I'll be working at the desk and things will fall on the floor, repeatedly. It's just, like, "Screw you." I just have to laugh at myself, because when I do that it makes me feel better and I get control back. I pick up the papers and think, "Hey, this is a game..." Really, you've got to play it as a game... "Someone's up there and they're messing with my head...."

It's all what you make of it, how you perceive it. You see, if I come across something that needs to be done, or that hinders me in any way, then I find a way that'll work. Rather than using a reacher, sometimes I can pick something up off the floor faster just by bending over and manipulating it just so. But a lot of people can't do that. I was blessed with long arms. It's all a matter of technique.

In the winter, Brian particularly enjoys using his long arms and technique for sit-skiing. This is a sport just like downhill skiing, except Brian is always in a seated position with his legs extended outward in front of him. Through an organization called Shared Adventures, Brian has access to a fiberglass sled with ski-like runners. He sits in the sled with poles taped to his hands and, tethered to an assistant, is able to downhill ski. He controls his skiing through the use of his poles and by shifting his body weight. With this adapted equipment, Brian is able to enjoy — and participate in — a sport we usually associate with strong leg muscles and agile movements.

During his other leisure hours, Brian goes out with friends. However, he feels he's grown away from his old friends and he says he'd like more opportunities to talk with someone about his "private feelings."

I especially wish I had a girlfriend. It would be all that much... more. It would definitely give me a better perspective. You know, where I could share things with her and she could share things with me. Right now I'm just me, myself, and I know someday it'll happen, it's just a matter of when. It'll happen, just like everything else happens. That's an experience I've learned.

Not too many people have their life planned out for them like I've planned it out for myself. You can't dwell on the past; you can't dwell on the future, but you can't let it go either.

I get depressed. I think, "I wish I could live a normal life" — but then I realize I do live a normal life. Even better than normal. I think, "I wish I could lead an active life" — but then I realize I do live an active life. At times I wish I could get out and frolic in the snow — but I do frolic in the snow, because I go skiing.

You have to plan for the future. That's one of the things that makes me want to get up in the morning... having something to shoot for.

TWO DIFFERENT PEOPLE, TWO DIFFERENT FUTURES?

Unlike Brian, Chuck cannot live an independent life. The level of Chuck's spinal cord injury and the fact that, unlike Brian, he has no voluntary control over the movements of his shoulders or arms, means that he needs more assistance than assistive devices alone can provide. Brian primarily utilizes assistive devices, whereas Chuck relies mostly on personal assistants. For example, Chuck requires the assistance of someone — a family member, friend or paid personal assistant — to get him out of bed and into his wheelchair in the morning and to help him get dressed and groomed. He also needs someone to prepare his breakfast. However, with the use of assistive devices, particularly the more complex and computerized ones, Chuck can ultimately be less dependent on others for many of his activities.

Since Chuck has paralysis below his shoulders, he uses a battery-powered wheelchair activated and controlled through a joystick extension and operated by his head movements. When Chuck wants to turn right, he places his head against a crescent-shaped bar that extends from one side of his head, around the back to the other side of his head, and applies pressure to that part of the bar near his right ear. When he gets to an elevator, he grabs his mouthstick with his teeth, sets it on the elevator button, and with a forward head movement presses the elevator button. Chuck's power wheelchair is an assistive technology device. It alone gives him control over much of the mobility lost in his motorcycle accident.

Chuck can have control over when his coffee is ready in the morning by using the same system designed for the general population — a coffeemaker with a timer that can be set the night before. It can be controlled by an environmental control system (ECS), also referred to as an electronic aid to daily living (EADL), customized especially for Chuck through the use of different types of switches. Depending on the amount of functioning and gross and fine movement a person has available, environmental control systems can be operated through a mouthstick, a puff-and-sip pneumatic control (for those with enough ventilatory control), or through a voice-activated mechanism. Each ECS or EADL has the capability to remotely control a variety of household appliances such as a coffeemaker, TV, radio, lights, automatic dialing telephones, and intercoms.

In the morning, Chuck could open the door for his personal assistant by using his ECS or EADL to release the front door lock. He could have the coffee ready so that his assistant just needed to pour it into the cup for him. Prototypes of robotic and expert systems have been developed to perform many of the routine functions done for individuals by their assistants.

Service animals (typically dogs, but also chimpanzees and monkeys) have been trained to perform some of these same functions. Service animals assist individuals in many ways. They are trained to fetch and return dropped or needed items and to pull wheelchairs up ramps or across distances that individuals with disabilities are incapable of attaining independently. Service animals have also been trained to do other tasks such as turning switches on and off, opening doors, carrying materials, handing in paperwork and mailing letters (Zapf, 1998a). While they have different capabilities than many assistive technologies, but less than a personal assistant, there is a lack of agreement in the disability community today about the advisability of having these animals as a primary contact rather than a human assistant. For many individuals, the care and attention demanded by a service animal is beyond their ability or desire to provide. For others, their service animals serve as important companions and "social magnets" or icebreakers, as people will approach them and talk about the animal whereas they might have avoided any contact otherwise. It is important to note that the Americans with Disabilities Act recognizes service animals as interventions for assisting people with disabilities (Zapf, 1998a). It is just as important to note that the match of person and service animal requires careful evaluation and training (Zapf, 1998b).

After Chuck's assistant helps him in grooming and dressing, he can either be fed by his assistant or eat his breakfast independently through the use of an automatic self-feeding device. Once his food is placed in a special ridged and sectioned plate, it is revolved to a certain point or setting where a spoon is attached to an arm slot control. When the plate has stopped in the preselected setting, the arm moves down to scoop up the food in the spoon, then raises it to mouth level so Chuck can have a portion of food. This isn't a fast process, but it does enable Chuck to enjoy independence in eating. It frees his assistant to work on something else for him.

After breakfast, Chuck requires help from a caretaker or personal assistant in cleaning the feeder and the kitchen in general. But once he's groomed, dressed, and fed, Chuck, too, could independently access his own van — using full head, not hand, controls. The differences in cost between a van for Chuck and Brian's van are great. Chuck's need for such devices as an automatic feeder and an environmental control system make the costs of his independence higher in general than Brian's. This applies to a work setting, too, because Chuck would not only need a specialized desk to accommodate his wheelchair, but would need all his work tools connected to a computer so that everything could be activated by his mouthstick or his voice. He could use a hands-free phone with a headset for privacy and an intercom system for communicating with coworkers. Computer diskettes could contain the materials he had to read or reference.

Workstations for higher-level tetraplegics like Chuck are quite sophisticated because users with such limited functional movements cannot access a large working area. However, items can be set on turntables (like Chuck's plate on his automatic self-feeder) that can be moved into an accessible position by the push of a computer button. With this done, Chuck's computer, like Brian's, can give him access to anyone, anywhere in the world.

As these examples show, high-tech products have been a boon in enabling individuals with physical disabilities to lead more independent lives. But their individual stories also highlight the fact that not all persons with disabilities can benefit equally from technology, and certainly not with identical amounts of financial resources. Chuck's assistive devices need to be more complex, and thus are often more expensive than Brian's. Also, while Brian can take advantage of newer high-tech devices, in some cases he can choose to use a simple reacher or, as he said earlier, to pick up an object off the floor "just by bending over and manipulating it just so." Chuck does not have as many options and would lead a much more restricted life than he does now if not for his personal assistants and assistive devices.

It is important to keep such distinctions in mind when comparing people's opinions of their assistive devices. At times Chuck gets irritated with his devices and focuses on their limitations and faults because he can exercise so few choices around their cost, level of technical sophistication, and even whether or not he can try to get along without them. And when he does use his devices, his social and recreational options cannot come close to those of someone like Brian. Brian, however, in spite of his many capabilities, also has bouts of dejection and shares Chuck's feelings of being restricted, especially in the area of intimate relationships.

CHAPTER TWO

Independent for the First Time

Success is counted sweetest
By those who ne'er succeed.
— EMILY DICKINSON

Chuck and Brian are just two examples of young adults with disabilities. Their present lives may seem restricted and incomplete compared to life before their injuries. Some individuals, however, who have had severe disabilities since birth or shortly thereafter, rarely had the opportunity to do *anything* on their own. Jim, born with cerebral palsy, was diagnosed as mentally retarded. His parents were advised to institutionalize him because he would need permanent custodial care. He learned to feed himself at 19 and to drive at 21. At 25, he was hired as an accountant for a major insurance company.

JIM, 1986

Jim, 34, has severe cerebral palsy (CP) that affects all his movements and involves his entire body. I knew from talking with him over the phone when arranging our meeting that his speech intelligibility is poor. Like many people with CP, he sounds like a tape played at too slow a speed. In addition, his words are ill-formed, as if spoken with a thick tongue. The speech muscles of many people with CP are weak and difficult to control.

Jim said it would be most convenient for us to meet in his office and that the best time would be from noon to one, during his lunch hour. He expressed a strong desire that our meeting should not interfere with his work time.

Jim works in the world headquarters of his company. The huge main floor of his building was filled with suited executives hurrying among live full-size trees, modern sculptures, and escalators. There was a constant din of indiscernible conversation buzzing by. Elevator bells were popping at the rate of an automatic weapon, each detonation bringing a corps of business infantrymen storming towards the yet unopened doors. The place was frenetic.

Jim had given me detailed directions to his office, but I really wasn't sure how to get there because I had been too reluctant to ask him to keep repeating the directions. I figured that once I got inside the building I'd either be able to figure it out for myself or find someone to direct me.

I got off the elevator on the fifth floor and felt relief at the contrasting quiet and calm. There wasn't a single person in sight, so I decided to turn right towards a set of closed doors that looked into a large area that appeared to be partitioned into office cubicles.

As soon as I was inside those doors a figure suddenly appeared and said, "Hi. You must be Marcia. I'm Jim's friend, Paul." His hand was waiting to shake mine and his smile was relaxed and warm in spite of his carefully crafted "dispassionate professional" image: three-piece suit, starched white shirt and broad-shouldered, straight-backed young executive posture. He said that Jim's office was just a few steps to our left. I noted it was the first office anyone would come to when entering that wing of Jim's department.

Jim was sitting at his desk waiting for me. An attractive man with long blond hair and classic features, he greeted me with friendly charm. He, too, was wearing a three-piece suit, but his ensemble included a brightly colored shirt with a pattern. It was obvious that Jim needed a shave, and the muscles in his mouth were weak so that when he spoke he drooled — which would cause Paul to come to his assistance with a tissue.

I recall trying to picture a Type-A business person meeting with Jim. How many people, I wondered, would feel comfortable working with Jim and would have the patience to listen to Jim's slow, slurred speech?

We stayed in Jim's office just long enough for him to show me the adapted equipment he uses to do his work. Other than a few low-tech modifications such as a modified computer keyboard and a telephone with oversize buttons, he went about his job tasks like any other accountant. I recall that his office was sparse in decor, and remember noticing only papers, reports, and computer printouts strewn about. He had a communication device to produce speech from words he typed into it, but told me he doesn't use it, because:

> ... around here, you have to keep up a fast pace. If you call and get a machine, what do you think? You usually hang up. Also, people don't want to take the time.

I didn't tell Jim that I find speech from a communication device preferable to not understanding — or misunderstanding — someone. I figured if there were any real problems, his supervisor would have made Jim aware of them by now.

Jim said that we had been given the use of a small room in the next wing for our meeting. He is ambulatory, but walking is a slow and physically strenuous process for him. Therefore, Jim often uses an electric scooter to give him speed in getting around the building. His scooter is a powered three-wheel vehicle with a chair and armrests. It has handlebars similar to those on a bicycle, and a bicycle-type basket to carry papers, printouts, his briefcase, and other items. For cross-town trips and for getting between his apartment and work, Jim drives his own fully equipped van.

We went down the corridor and into the next wing. We passed several of his colleagues who either acknowledged us with a smile and a head nod, a greeting, or a joke. Later, Jim asked me,

> **J:**   At your job, when you walk down the halls, does everyone keep talking to you all the time like that?
>
> **M:**   I don't know... I guess so, Jim. What do you mean?
>
> **J:**   Well, a lot of times I'll be trying to concentrate on something, I'll be deep in thought, and they'll interrupt me. Is it just me, or does everyone have that?

Jim wanted reassurance that he was truly being greeted as a colleague and not as a "handicapped person in need of cheery pick-me-ups all the time."

Once we were in the next wing, a secretary met us with the news that Jim's supervisor had given us the use of the conference room for the rest of the afternoon, "if we so wished." I recall being surprised and puzzled by this: What happened to the strict "one-hour lunch break" interview? And why? I wondered if Jim's supervisor considered him as professional as he believed himself to be.

The conference room was one of those plush, soundproof rooms adorned with whiteboards, spare writing tablets, and continuous coffee service. It was a wonderfully luxurious place in which to talk, but totally unnecessary, maybe even inappropriate, and much too large for just Jim and me. At Jim's suggestion, we helped ourselves to coffee, picked two of the upholstered chairs at one end of the table and settled into a corner of the room that we were able to make seem rather cozy. Jim and I talked for the next two hours. While I often had to ask him to repeat things for me, I gradually got accustomed to his communication style and, with benefit of his facial expressions and body language, had less and less trouble understanding him.

I'm the youngest of four kids. When I was one year old, the doctor told my parents to institutionalize me because I'd never walk or talk, would never know anything. It wasn't until I was 17 that they finally realized I wasn't retarded.

But my mother knew all along I wasn't retarded and my parents refused to put me in an institution. I got speech, occupational, and physical therapy and I was able to crawl. Doctors added weights to my body, which I carried around during the day, to slow my jerky movements and build up my muscles. I had wheels on my first walker, and once I'd get going I'd make that thing fly. Eventually, they took the wheels off.

I went to a school for the handicapped from when I was 6 to when I was 17. When I was working in a sheltered workshop, they had me supervising other people. But they were paying me the same sheltered workshop wages.

Because of his poor speech intelligibility, Jim's bright mind wasn't discovered until he was 17. As he sees it,

Society looks at people who are blind or who use crutches and does not consider them to be mentally retarded. But they label people who have speech problems as mentally retarded.

When he was 17, Jim could not yet read or write, and he was placed in special education classes at his local high school. After just a few months, however, he was placed in regular classes because "Special Ed was just too easy."

After graduating from high school, Jim enrolled in a community college. Still unable to read, the frustrations of college landed him in the hospital. It was then that rehabilitation professionals got involved.

I went into rehabilitation to learn to drive, but they said I first had to learn to feed myself. I resisted it, but in two weeks I was able to feed myself. They discovered that even though I'm right-handed, my left hand works better for feeding.

I really came to believe that I can do the same things as everyone else, even though I may need more time. I learned to walk unaided at 10, to read and feed myself at 19 and to drive a vehicle at 21. Maybe I learned later than most people how to do these things, but I did learn.

Rehabilitation gave me a tutor for reading and taught me how to drive. I dropped out of college, but I enrolled in a special program for the handicapped. Then I enrolled in another college for a degree in accounting.

Jim was one of thirty "handicapped but bright" individuals selected over a five-year time span for a special career training program that placed individuals for a year-long trial with appropriate employers. That was how Jim found his way to the insurance company, where he's been for the past four years.

> This is a big step in my life... the final stretch of fitting into the career world. Walking out of the building with a suit on and carrying my work... and I'm just beginning.

I went back to Jim's office with him. As I was putting on my coat, Jim motioned for me to sit down and said,

> You know, there were four of us boys basically alike at age 7. We were inseparable. One of them has died because he gave up. He got pneumonia from not wearing the right clothes for cold weather. Two are in sheltered workshops — and one of them can't handle his own finances and needs people to do everything for him.

I asked, "What do you think it is, Jim, that makes you so different from those other guys?"
He didn't have to think a second for his answer.

> Encouragement... and courage. I was afraid I'd be alone someday. I have two parents and a brother and two sisters who would do anything for me, but they have their own lives. My parents treated us all the same and gave us a lot of encouragement. Once, to motivate me to be independent, they said, 'Hey, someday we're not going to be here.' That is reality.
> I'm very glad I have my scooter and my van and my other aids. When you have a handicap, you need to find a new way of doing what you can't do by yourself. Parents and other caretakers will pass away. And there's a difference in being dependent on people or devices. People may or may not be there when you need them, but devices are still in the place where you last used them.
> It's such a shame that...

Jim suddenly looked tired and there was a sadness in his eyes I hadn't seen before.

> ...that... well, devices don't have expectations, but people can have expectations that can hold you back.

CEREBRAL PALSY: DEMOGRAPHICS, PHYSICAL EFFECTS, AND FUNCTIONAL EXPECTATIONS

As with a spinal cord injury, a person with severe cerebral palsy can have a lifelong limitation in mobility. Cerebral palsy (CP) also results from injury — not to the spinal cord, but to the brain either before, during, or after birth. The causes of cerebral palsy include illness during pregnancy, premature delivery, or lack of oxygen supply to the baby; or it may occur early in life as a result of an accident, lead poisoning, viral infection, child abuse, or other factors.[1] Put together, the words cerebral (meaning "brain") and palsy ("motor disability") provide a verbal description of CP as a motor disability caused by a dysfunction in the brain. There are many different types of CP that vary according to the particular type of motor dysfunction: e.g., spasticity, athetosis, ataxia. There are approximately 500,000-700,000 people in the U.S. who have CP and there are approximately 5,000 babies and infants diagnosed with CP each year with another 1,500 or so acquiring a diagnosis of CP in the early years of life.

Like spinal cord injuries, cerebral palsy can drastically reduce or totally curtail mobility and physical movements. But while people with CP and spinal cord injuries can share similar mobility disabilities, cerebral palsy is a group of conditions. People with CP often have additional impairments, because cerebral palsy affects people in a wider variety of ways than spinal cord injuries do. As described by William Rush (1985), who has CP himself: "[CP] can leave a person with only a slight limp or it can leave a person unable to walk, talk, see and hear... [D]epending on the location and severity of the damage, cerebral palsy can also leave a person mentally competent or mentally retarded" (p. 27). Like a spinal cord injury, however, "it is not inherited, contagious, or terminal."

Dale Baum noted in his 1992 book, *The Human Side of Exceptionality*:

> For every 100,000 people born in one year, seven will have cerebral palsy. Of these seven: 1 will die in infancy, 2 of the remaining 6 will be mentally retarded and will require permanent custodial care, the remaining 4 will require medical and habilitation services, and finally, out of this group 1 may go to college. (p. 181)

While the above statistical breakdown may be out of date, it is interesting that Jim gave a similar breakdown on page 24 for himself and his three seven-year-old friends.

Cerebral palsy is a developmental disability. The Developmental Disabilities Assistance and Bill of Rights Amendments of 2000 (PL 106-402), which is commonly referred to as the "DD Act" or "Developmental Disabilities Act" defines a developmental disability as a severe, chronic disability of an individual 5 years of age or older which:

(A) is attributable to a mental or physical impairment or combination of mental and physical impairments;
(B) is manifested before the individual attains age 22;
(C) is likely to continue indefinitely;
(D) results in substantial functional limitations in three or more of the following areas of major life activity —
   (i) self-care;
   (ii) receptive and expressive language;
   (iii) learning;
   (iv) mobility;
   (v) self-direction;
   (vi) capacity for independent living; and
   (vii) economic self-sufficiency; and
(E) reflects the individual's need for a combination and sequence of special, interdisciplinary, or generic services, supports, or other assistance that is of lifelong or extended duration and is individually planned and coordinated, except that such term, when applied to infants and young children means individuals from birth to age 5, inclusive, who have substantial developmental delay or specific congenital or acquired conditions with a high probability of resulting in developmental disabilities if services are not provided.

In addition to cerebral palsy, developmental disabilities include mental retardation, Down syndrome, epilepsy, autism, chronic illness and sensory impairment.

Many Differences Can Exist Between Acquired and Congenital Disabilities

Jim's life history illustrates a major difference between a person born with a *congenital disability*, like cerebral palsy, and someone like Chuck or Brian who acquired a disability in adulthood (known as having an *acquired disability*). Jim sees his assistive devices as having opened entirely new worlds to him and as keys to new experiences, opportunities and independence that would not have been possible without them. Jim has only experienced newfound capabilities. Unlike Chuck or Brian, he has not experienced sudden functional loss with only a portion of previous functioning regained through the use of assistive technologies. When Jim goes into a restaurant with his friends from work, his feelings are very different from those of Chuck, who was accustomed to walking in with friends before his accident and now feels patronized when he accompanies them in restaurants. Even though Brian is grateful for his van and being back on the road again, his gratitude doesn't compare to Jim's awe at being able to drive himself to and from work.

While Chuck and Brian also highly prize opportunity, independence, and new experiences, their assistive technologies represent compensation for what they can no longer do themselves. For them, a simple, low-tech device becomes a status symbol because it signifies both capability and ingenuity. Jim and other people with CP who use sophisticated high-tech devices, however, are usually perceived as having higher cognitive capabilities than CP users of simpler, low-tech, devices. Part of the status of high-tech device use comes from the belief that the CP user must be unusually endowed with financial resources and intelligence. In fact, in 1986, the typical adult with CP lacked the social or educational background to take advantage of the opportunities of high-tech assistance and often appeared under-educated and unsophisticated when compared to more advantaged peers — or to the person with an acquired disability who experienced a so-called normal educational process.

Maggie provides an example of the value of some of the newer, high-tech devices for the older person with CP who has been educationally and socially advantaged. Because of her communication system and a growing consumer empowerment movement, she had social and job opportunities in 1986 that she never believed she would have.

MAGGIE, 1986

I had been traveling and interviewing people all day. Feeling tired both emotionally and physically, the only thing I was thinking about was a quiet evening alone. However, when I reached my hotel room, I noticed the message light on my phone flashing. The message was from Maggie, a person in training for a new computerized communication device whom I was scheduled to interview the next day at the rehabilitation center. She was inquiring if we might meet that night at her mother's friend's apartment, since the next day she had to go apartment hunting and wouldn't be at the rehabilitation center. She left the phone number where she was staying and suggested a meeting time of 7 o'clock.

I looked at the clock and saw it was already 6:30 — where had the time gone? My decision was made instantly: If I didn't meet with Maggie tonight, chances were we wouldn't be able to get together again before I had to fly back. It was either tonight or not at all, and not-at-all was out of the question.

I called to confirm our meeting and found out that Maggie had just been offered a job in another town, hence her need to go apartment hunting. With a degree in social work, she was about to become a community services coordinator for an Independent Living Center. I ran a brush through my hair and headed outside to catch a cab. Twenty minutes later I was there.

As soon as I walked into the apartment I saw Maggie sitting in a battery-powered wheelchair so large it overpowered the apartment's living room. She was very excited about her job offer, and her excitement made her spasticity very evident. Maggie struggled to speak, but the end result of all her effort was a string of wordless sounds only decipherable by those familiar with her particular speech patterns.

Maggie's mother and her friend were there, as well as Maggie's companion and assistant, Theresa. Maggie and Theresa met several years before in a sheltered workshop. Theresa had been institutionalized for most of her life because of Down syndrome,[2] yet she drives, does all of the cooking, and is a good assistant for Maggie. While Maggie is very intelligent and has a college degree, she is extremely limited physically. Thus, she and Theresa have capabilities which complement one another so that the needs of both are well met.

Maggie, 42, with severe (athetoid) cerebral palsy, has total-body involvement and no discernible unaided speech. She communicates by using a manual communication board and is in the process of learning to use the Express III (computerized) communication system at the rehabilitation center.

Maggie's manual board is a very basic one featuring individual boxes with each letter of the alphabet, the numbers 0-9, and such key phrases as "Please," "Thank you," "I want," etc. Manual communication boards are highly individualized. Speech therapists adapt them to each individual's communication preferences. While Maggie's board contains letters, numbers, and phrases, boards for nonverbal children or illiterate adults may have pictures or use the international Blissymbolics.[3] A manual communication board user, or sender, points to a symbol (a letter, word, number or picture) with a finger or some other type of pointer. The custom followed by receivers is to repeat out loud the entire message as it has been understood. This tells the board user that the message has or has not been understood accurately. With an affirmative head nod, the user acknowledges accurate understanding. A negative head nod immediately followed by continued pointing indicates clarification is in process.

I had hoped to see Maggie's Express III in action, and was disappointed to learn she was keeping it at the rehabilitation center during her training. Thus, her means of communication tonight was to be the manual board.

The use of a manual communication board is tedious for both the user and receiver, as I was to experience that evening with Maggie. The temptation is always great for the parent or friend to jump in and finish sentences for the belabored speaker. Maggie, in order to prevent just such a thing from happening, had asked to meet with me alone so that her responses wouldn't be "interpreted," as she put it. However, all five of us ended up sitting around the kitchen table, and for three hours we watched Maggie slowly and arduously spell out her responses to my questions, seeing her resort to abbreviations and shorthand ways of getting her message across.

A typical exchange would go something like this:

"Tell me, Maggie, what is the biggest advantage of the Express III over this board?"

"They have voice in computer."

When I asked Maggie for her definition of a "rehabilitation success" she replied: "Me."

Further probing led into her perception of her quality of life, which she described as: "Good because I am determined."

"Is there anything that would make it better?"

"I would like more of a social life."

After a short break for cake and coffee, we resumed our slow conversation. Towards the end, Maggie's obvious physical exhaustion, coupled with everyone's general fatigue, caused all of us to jump in and try to finish Maggie's words and thoughts for her. It was becoming a game of "Twenty Questions," but Maggie didn't even mind anymore. Thus it was obviously time to end the interview.

Without a background of quality social and educational experiences, many adults in 1986 who had been born with disabilities (those with cerebral palsy being just one example) would not have the same opportunities as Maggie. Then and now they often live at or below the poverty line, and their lack of financial resources — together with their lack of sophistication about high-tech assistive devices — results in situations where they not only can't afford devices, but might not understand the fundamentals of their operation without considerable training (which is also expensive). Thus, they can very easily become stuck in a state of perpetual and permanent deprivation.

While today is an especially exciting time for children with cerebral palsy, the person with a developmental disability who in 1986 was 30 years of age or older represented a transition between two worlds: the pre-technology and pre-civil rights world of relative segregation and deprivation, and the high-tech world of enhanced capabilities and newly gained opportunities. Traversing through such a transition was often difficult — for some, even perilous.

BASIC FACTS ABOUT THE PEOPLE IN THIS BOOK

In Table 2-1 on the following page, a summary lists key characteristics of the individuals who share their experiences and perspectives in this book. This will be a useful reference as their life examples continue to evolve through the next eight chapters.

Footnotes Chapter 2

[1] Cerebral palsy is characterized according to the type and extent of motor involvement. The March of Dimes website [http://www.marchofdimes.com/professionals/681_1208.asp] defines three types:

    a. *Spasticity.* Spasticity is the most common type of cerebral palsy. It is found in about 70 to 80 % of cases, mostly with hemiplegia (paralysis of one side of the body) or less likely, with tetraplegia (total paralysis of the body from the neck down). The muscle tone is increased, and there is increased resistance to passive movement. When the muscles are stretched, as in attention to movement, there is an increased stretch reflex and the muscle contracts strongly, involuntarily and inaccurately. The person walks with a characteristic "scissor gait."

    b. *Athetosis.* Athetosis is a type of cerebral palsy found in approximately 10 to 20 % of people with CP. Purposeful movements are contorted and the person has abnormal posturing and uncontrollable and uncoordinated jerky, twisting movements of the extremities. The head is often drawn back with the mouth open. In trying to talk, the person may grimace. Walking may vary according to circumstances, perhaps improving when the person is not anxious and is well rested.

    c. *Ataxia.* This is a rather uncommon type of cerebral palsy, varying between 5-10 % of the population of persons with CP. The person has a disturbed sense of balance and has a greatly decreased capability for maintaining balance or coordination. The person may exhibit a high stepping gait and may stumble, lurch and fall easily. Nystagmus (involuntary rapid eye movement) and tremor of the head may be seen.

    Many individuals with severe CP have a combination of the above characteristics.

[2] In 1854, Dr. Langdon Down described a certain group of people according to the following common characteristics: eyes that slope at the outer corners, the impression of a broad flat face, small stubby hands, shorter physique and smaller head. People with Down syndrome look so similar to one another that it seems they must all be siblings. The majority of individuals with Down syndrome are at least slightly retarded. In 1959, it was discovered that the cause of Down syndrome is an extra chromosome — 47 instead of the normal 46.

[3] A system composed of over 2,000 graphic symbols that can be combined and recombined in endless ways to create new symbols and has the potential to facilitate international communication over the Internet. Further information can be obtained at http://home.istar.ca/~bci/

Table 2-1: Brief Biographical Summary of the People in This Book

	ACQUIRED SPINAL CORD INJURIES IN ADULTHOOD			
	Ken	Brian	Chuck	Butch
TYPE OF INJURY	C6 complete SCI at age 18 from a fall	C6 complete SCI at age 17 from a motorcycle accident	C4 complete SCI at age 29 from a motorcycle accident	C7-8 complete SCI from an automobile accident
AGE IN 1996	40 (22 years post-injury)	35 (18 years post-injury)	43 (14 years post-injury)	46 (14 years post-injury)
DEVICES USED	Power wheelchair, van	Power wheelchair, van	Power wheelchair	Power wheelchair (with hydraulic lift)
LIVING STATUS	County Hospital, then apartments Died 09/95	Parents' home, then moved to California	Sister's home in rural area Died in 2003	Parents' home Died 03/99
WORK STATUS	Social worker; counselor for an Independent Living Center Dropped out of graduate program	Engineering degree, several jobs, many recreational interests of high risk	Former bartender	Former garbage truck driver

	BORN WITH CEREBRAL PALSY			
	Jim	Maggie	Ann	Linda
AGE IN 1996	41	52	57	67
DEVICES USED	Electric scooter, van	Power wheelchair, augmentative communication device	Manual, then power wheelchair; wordboard	Power wheelchair
LIVING STATUS	Condo, then apartment	Apartment with caregiver	Nursing home, then apartment	
WORK STATUS	Accountant	Terminated from job as Community Services Coordinator for an Independent Living Center	None	

CHAPTER THREE

Assistive Technologies as "World-Openers"

> *Between two worlds life hovers like a star,*
> *'Twixt night and morn, upon the horizon's verge.*
> *How little do we know that which we are!*
> *How less what we may be!*
>
> — BYRON

ASSISTANCE COMES IN MANY FORMS

Christopher Nolan, an Irish poet and author who has cerebral palsy, cannot produce intelligible sounds or walk; he only has voluntary control over nodding his head. In his autobiography (1987), he describes how he felt being able to use a typewriter at age 11 to express his thoughts and ideas. With his mother steadying his head so that he could apply a pointer to the typewriter keyboard, he "typed beauty from within, beauty of secret knowledge so secretly hidden and so nearly lost forever" (Nolan, 1987, p. 56). Some years later, a computer scientist worked with him on the use of a word processor. Nolan describes his experience as follows:

> With the alphabet upon the screen and the cursor hopping along from one letter to the next, all [I] had to do now was strike [my] chin against a nearby placed switch and miracle of miracles, the letter would appear in a boxed-off area of the screen. There and then disability would be conquered. Conscious of the greatness in that movement by which [I] struck the chin-switch, [I] waited for the green cursor to come to the required letter, but by that time [my] acute mind had foreseen the difficulty, [my] entire body froze rigid, and [my] eyes watched the cursor hop by... The next time was the same and the next... [On the next attempt I] made a wallop at the switch which almost beheaded me... (p. 83-84).

The experiences of Christopher Nolan, Jim, and Maggie (as well as countless unnamed others) highlight the fact that, without the means to access communication devices, typewriters or word processors, a brilliant mind can be a secret "nearly lost forever." However, as happened with Christopher Nolan, each individual finds that one or more of the available options are more productive and work better than others. Hence, users need to have a choice among options.

Computer technology may not be the most efficient answer for all individuals with severe cerebral palsy. Christopher Nolan had been doing very well with the typewriter as long as he had someone to steady his head. He tried a word processor, but gave up using it. Jim, too, prefers not to use his communication device. He believes it is "inefficient" as it does not allow him to keep up with the fast pace around his office. Maggie, who is like Christopher Nolan in that she has no articulate speech, is unlike him in that she has chosen to try to master the use of a computerized device.

Computerized communication devices are a much more complex and sophisticated means of communication than Maggie's manual communication board, described in Chapter Two. Computers require considerable training and are expensive. Users need to have a fondness for computers, the cognitive abilities to operate a computer, and a tolerance for speech output that does not sound particularly natural. They must also have the patience to communicate according to the machine's pace and its manner of constructing messages. Many devices are underused in natural environments because users find it difficult to go with a natural conversation flow and find use fatiguing. To give readers a sense of these factors, a description follows of the Express I, the first member of Prentke Romich Company's Express family of "augmentative communication devices" — devices used to augment the available communication skills of a person with a speech disability. The Express III that Maggie is in the process of learning differs from the Express I primarily in its synthesized voice output quality.

> It is a small computer activated by one of a variety of switches (a joystick, a mouthstick, an arm-slot control, a manual pointer, an optical headpointer) and through any part of the body the user can control — head, tongue, chin, shoulder, knee, even a puff of breath. "Direct selection" can be gained to all the board's capabilities by directly touching a square on the board's matrix with a finger or a pointer. Indirect access can be accomplished with a joystick that remotely controls a light spot on the board which scans in any direction until the desired square is reached. The joystick method takes a little longer, but it accomplishes the task with no more than gross movement.
>
> The slowest process, again providing indirect access to the board, is "row-column scanning" accessed by paddle, wobble or puff/sip switches. The operator hits the switch once to make the scanner start. The light spot then goes line by line until the operator makes it stop at the desired square by hitting the switch again.

The Express can store on four different levels the same kinds of words, phrases and symbols used on a manual board. Once the user accesses a square, the selection appears in a display box at the top of the device. Spelling or wording can be changed, and words can be connected into sentences before they are printed out or spoken through the voice synthesizer.

The Express III is designed to accept a wide variety of peripherals and attachments such as a video display for a television screen, an automatic telephone, and, through an environmental control system, any electrical appliance. It can be connected to a personal computer and, thus, to all of the workday and leisure applications a computer offers. Since the Express III became available, the fundamentals of augmentative communication devices have changed very little. Efforts have primarily focused on ways to enhance the speed of the device without adding complexity to its use.

The choices available today for communication — from gestures to wordboards to computerized devices that speak for the person — are nothing short of a major revolution. Today, the mind of a child born with cerebral palsy who cannot speak is not apt to be a mind "nearly lost forever." That child will go to school and will be a visible member of the adult community.

To have a sense of the revolution assistive technology has brought about, compare Jim's life with that of Jeremiah (Lange, 1995). Jeremiah was about 6 years old when his occupational therapist first started to work with him. He has spastic tetraplegia from cerebral palsy, and

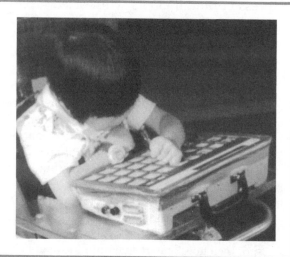

**Figure 3-1:
An electronic
communication
device in use**

*Photo courtesy of the
Center for Assistive
Technology, Dept. of
Occupational Therapy,
University at Buffalo*

average intelligence. He also has low vision. Born in 1979, Jeremiah was using an Apple computer in preschool. Born in 1952, Jim's parents were advised to institutionalize him.

Jeremiah received his first computerized communication device and power wheelchair when he was 9 years old. By the time he started high school, Jeremiah had already presented a speech on technology before the governor of Colorado. By contrast, at 16, Jim could not yet feed himself. While it is true that Jim is functioning at a high level today, and that "maybe I learned later than most people how to do these things, but I did learn," he spent many frustrating years trying to convince people of his capabilities — frustrations that have left permanent scars on his psyche and identity.

Gordon Richmond, 35, relates the changes he has experienced over the years because of assistive technology:

> Before technology entered my life, I, like many others, was trapped within myself. I didn't have transportation. I didn't have a job to support myself. Most of all, I did not have a good way to express my thoughts and feelings. It is now through technology that I have a service that transports me. It is now through technology that I have not just a job but a career to use my capabilities to the fullest. It is now through technology that I have an effective and articulate way of expressing my thoughts and feelings (Richmond, 1996).

In Chapter One, Brian said how grateful he is for his assistive technologies. Without them, he would not be able to live the independent lifestyle he enjoys. Because of his power wheelchair and van, he has the mobility to go just about anywhere he wishes.

Cody illustrates the differences technology can make in the life of a child with a spinal cord injury today. Cody received a C1-level spinal cord injury in an automobile accident in 1994, when he was six years old. Just twenty years ago, it is unlikely Cody would have survived his injuries. Today, he attends his local public school. He will thrive thanks to his power wheelchair, a computer that he controls with a mouthstick, and other assistive technologies.

Assistive technologies cover a broad range of devices for a broad range of functions. The growth in assistive technologies has been enormous. In 1969, 6.2 million people used a total of 7.2 million assistive devices. With the advent of the microcomputer in the late 1970s, the number of devices has multiplied dramatically. So, too, have the numbers of Americans using them. In 1990, more than 13 million people used assistive devices; yet more than 2.5 million persons needed devices they could not obtain, primarily because they could not afford them

(LaPlante, Hendershot, & Moss, 1992). While each passing half-decade has seen the quantity of assistive technologies in use increase markedly, the funding of these technologies is often complex and uncertain, and this situation is not apt to change in the near future. This topic will be discussed at greater length in Chapter Ten.

What Are Assistive Technologies?

Assistive technologies or devices are tools for enhancing the independent functioning of people who have physical limitations or disabilities. An assistive technology device, as defined in the "Technology-Related Assistance of Individuals with Disabilities Act of 1988" (P.L. 100-407), is

> any item, piece of equipment, or product system, whether acquired commercially off the shelf, modified or customized, that is used to increase, maintain, or improve functional capabilities of individuals with disabilities.

This definition of assistive devices has been used in each piece of legislation related to persons with disabilities passed since 1988 and it is the standard definition used in the field internationally.

Assistive devices are really just what the term implies — they assist individuals in performing certain functions like getting around in wheelchairs and in specially designed vans. *Adapted equipment* refers to devices designed for the general population, which are adapted in ways to be useful for people with disabilities (for example, telephones with a button to adjust the volume, ball ramps and bumpers for bowling lanes). Some adapted devices are so widely used and accepted that we don't think of them as adapted equipment at all. For example, an adapted equipment specialist for the United Cerebral Palsy Association in Rochester, NY, noted:

> We all use adapted equipment. Take for example the pencil I'm holding. It allows ideas in my brain to be recorded on paper. But millions and millions of people cannot use this pencil; generally they're in the first grade. So what do we do? We make larger pencils for them that they can hold. We give them a piece of adapted equipment. If there's enough people who can't use something, it will be adapted.

The distinctions between these terms are far from pure. The point is that without assistive devices made possible by relatively low-cost electronic components and computers, many people with physical disabilities would be leading isolated and dependent lives. As indicated in Chapter 1, today a person with functional movement of the arms and shoulders and above (C6 or lower spinal cord injuries) can live alone, travel, and work in a competitive job due to advances in technology. As recently as the early 1960s, most equipment available to individuals with disabilities was primarily of a mechanical nature. Wheelchairs were literally chairs on wheels. Prosthetic limbs were plastic or, earlier, metal and wooden replacements for lost arms or legs. Now, advances in electronics have made possible such products as environmental control systems; additional advances in materials (plastics, stainless aluminum, etc.) have made other devices more lightweight, portable, flexible and durable.

Assistive devices range from low-tech aids such as built-up handles on eating utensils to the high-tech, computerized communication systems used by Jeremiah and Maggie and the battery powered wheelchairs used by Brian, Chuck, Maggie and Cody. When people speak of *high-tech* assistive devices, assistive technologies, or rehabilitation technologies they are usually referring to those with electronic components or which are powered by a computer. The number of these devices has increased dramatically in recent years.

Devices that consist of non-mechanical adaptations to existing products (such as a special grip added to a pencil or pen) are called *low-tech or simple* devices. Those with simple mechanical operations can be considered to be "medium-tech." It is important to realize that by law all of these devices are *assistive technologies* and that a low-tech device has as much value as a high-tech one for users who find the device has enhanced their functioning, independence, and quality of life, as the examples of Chuck and Brian indicated in Chapter 1. It can generally be said that individuals with the most severe disabilities require the most customized and computerized technologies to enable their independent functioning. In fact, if these technologies were not available, many individuals would not be able to live independently in the community.

Purpose for Use of an Assistive Device

There are a number of ways to look at assistive devices. Here, devices are categorized by their purpose according to the resource book by Galvin and Scherer (1996).

A. Personal and self-care devices enable independence in such fundamental areas as grooming, bathing, dressing, eating and accessing home appliances. Low-tech options include nonslip placemats under dinner plates to prevent sliding of the plate, eating utensils that are angled or have a larger surface area for gripping, long handled

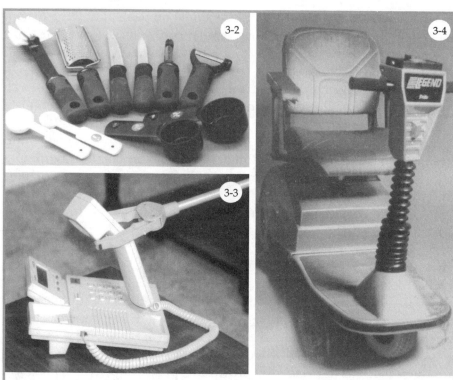

Figure 3-2: *Low-tech* – adapted cooking utensils with built-up handles for an easier grip.

Figure 3-3: *Medium-tech* – use of a reacher to pick up a telephone receiver.

Figure 3-4: *High-tech* – a powered scooter.

All photos courtesy of the Center for Assistive Technology, Department of Occupational Therapy, University at Buffalo.

sponges strapped across the back of the hand for bathing, Velcro closures instead of buttons on clothing, and special holders for pots and pans on the stove. Medium-and high-tech devices range from lamps that turn on and off by touching them anywhere on their base to complex environmental control systems that allow several appliances to be controlled by means of voice or through the use of such objects as a mouthstick. A mouthstick is a stick held between the teeth that can be used for pressing buttons, dialing phones, etc. It is not itself high-tech, but it provides a means of controlling many high-tech devices. These devices are most suitable for persons with functional limitations in the fingers, hands, and arms.

B. *Seating and mobility aids* include manual and battery-powered wheelchairs and scooters, wheelchair cushions, and accessories such as desktop-type boards for holding things, as well as backpacks and baskets for storage.

C. *Transportation aids* are for adapting vans and cars, including wheelchair lifts, hand controls, and wheelchair carriers. (A description of Brian's fully equipped van appeared in Chapter One.)

D. *Communication systems and devices* range from manual communication boards to computerized devices with synthesized speech output (such as the earlier generation device (Express) described in the previous chapter).

E. *Technologies for blindness and low vision* are for reading and for safe travel. Magnifiers, Braille or voice output systems for reading, and canes for travel are examples of devices in this category.

F. *Technologies for people who are hard-of-hearing or deaf* are for sound amplification (hearing aids, personal FM systems), access to information (captioned television, telephones which send text messages over telephone lines), and alerting or signaling (vibrotactile pagers, flashing timers and alarms). The American with Disabilities Act requires that telecommunication relay services operate 24 hours per day, seven days per week. This enables persons using a TTY (a type of machine that allows people with hearing or speech disabilities to communicate over the phone using a keyboard and a viewing screen) to communicate with hearing communication partners even though the latter do not have TTY access. A relay operator speaks the text typed by a deaf person, and types the speech of the hearing telephone partner that then appears on the deaf person's TTY. The Access Board, U.S. Architectural and Transportation Barriers Compliance Board, has an on-line guide on *Using a TTY available at*: http://www.access-board.gov/publications/UsingATTY/A2.html.

Devices may also be categorized according to the activities and environments they make accessible.

A. *Leisure and recreation.* Assistive devices have made most sports, recreational, and leisure activities accessible to persons with disabilities — from tethered sit-skiing to scuba diving, wheelchair basketball, sailing and card-shuffling.

B. *Child's play.* Adapted toys and do-it-yourself playthings for children are important assistive devices.

C. *Home and worksite.* Devices in this group focus on making the home and worksite accessible to the person with a disability. Such devices include workstations and adapted tools or appliances, as well as desirable modifications in these environments that allow for safe and easy movement.

Matching Devices to the Functional Limitations of the User

One can categorize devices in many different ways, including which functional limitations they address for the user.

Assistive devices for persons with functional limitations in the fingers, hands and arms. Many devices mentioned for helping with activities of daily living (see section A on page 39) can be useful in these areas. Telephones with speakerphone and abbreviated or quick-dialing capabilities are options that give persons with upper extremity limitations independence in calling and talking with other persons. A person with controllable movement of only the head can independently communicate on the telephone and turn appliances on and off. Thus, individuals paralyzed from the neck down, as well as those experiencing only weakness in one hand, have an array of options available to them. The major differences are that a person with *paralysis* will generally require the technology to do more and to be higher-tech than a person with hand *weakness.*

Table 3-1: Assistive devices for persons with functional limitations in the fingers, hands and arms

Extent of Functional Limitation	Complexity of Assistive Devices for Daily Living		
	Low-tech	*Medium-tech*	*High-tech*
mild	adapted eating utensils, bath sponge, non-slip placemat		
moderate		touch lamp	adapted telephones
severe			environmental control devices

Assistive devices for mobility for persons with functional limitations in the back, hips and legs. Technologies for mobility have made great strides, so that within each type of mobility-related device the user can also select from a number of options.

To be mobile is to be able to get around in one's environments and to exercise choice over the environments one wishes to be in. Low-tech products to facilitate mobility include basic canes and crutches. Canes can be made of wood or metal and can have a single foot or three or four "feet." A cane with four feet is referred to as a *quad cane*. They are useful for persons with weakness who desire assistance with their balance while walking.

Table 3-2: Assistive devices for mobility for persons with functional limitations in the back, hips and legs.

Extent of Functional Limitation	Complexity of Assistive Devices for Mobility		
	Low-tech	*Medium-tech*	*High-tech*
mild	single-foot cane, axillary crutch		
moderate		forearm crutches, rolling walkers, manual wheelchairs	manual wheelchairs with add-on power systems
severe			powered wheelchairs and scooters

Crutches, too, can be made of wood or metal. *Axillary crutches* support the person under the arm and require the hand to grip the crutch at around hip level. A *forearm crutch* has a cuff that goes around the arm to assist persons who do not have the hand strength for the use of an axillary crutch. These devices are more complex in design because they need to make up for more functional limitation. Another name for forearm crutches is "Lofstrand crutches."

Like canes and crutches, *walkers* come in several styles depending on the person's functional need and preferences. Basically, a walker is a lightweight three-sided frame that extends in front and on both sides of the person. Although walkers come in a variety of sizes and shapes and have many different features, they all have four points of contact with the floor or ground. Walkers are usually adjustable in height so that the top is slightly below the user's waist, enabling the person to lean on it for support and balance while walking. A walker provides a wide base of support. It may have wheels, which are helpful on cement or linoleum, but not as useful on carpeting.

Wheelchairs are used by persons who cannot walk unassisted and, thus, need more assistance with mobility than can be obtained from a walker. Wheelchairs are "chairs on wheels" and they are either manual (the wheels are manually propelled or rotated by the user or someone pushes the wheelchair for the user) or battery-powered or motorized. A joystick, a sip-and-puff tube, or a voice-activated interface controls the speed and direction of powered wheelchairs. Individuals using wheelchairs may need to have additional devices or products to ensure their comfort and safety. These include such things as tilt and recline features on the wheelchair itself, or special support cushions. Optional equipment may involve adding a hydraulic mechanism to raise and lower the wheelchair seat, and such accessories as wheelchair back-packs, baskets, lap trays and cup holders. Powered wheelchair and powered scooter users also require ramps for accessing different levels of buildings, and lifts for getting into vans and buses independently. Both manual and powered wheelchairs require special tie-down and restraint systems while riding in other vehicles such as buses or vans. A person using a powered wheelchair who wishes to drive typically needs to have a van equipped with hand or head controls.

Limitations in mobility are associated with limitations in such functions as reaching objects in high places or located at a distance from the user. *Reachers* are devices used to grab objects from a distance of approximately three feet from the user. One type is the pistol-grip reach-er that opens and shuts a two-pronged gripper on the end by activating a trigger on the handle.

The burgeoning growth of assistive technologies has formed a new industry. There are manufacturers devoted to their production and professional specializations to their selection and provision. The history of this development against the backdrop of the social and cultural treatment of individuals with disabilities over time is the substance of the next chapter.

FOR MORE INFORMATION

There are hundreds of products within each of the categories mentioned here. To obtain more detailed information about assistive technology devices, check the Yellow Pages under the headings "Medical Equipment and Supplies" and "Hospital Equipment and Supplies."

A visit to a dealer/supplier will show the very wide range of options available in devices for mobility, daily activities, self-care, etc. These businesses often have a person on staff who advises people on equipment and can help secure funding. Many dealers/suppliers may also supply devices on a loan or rental basis so individuals can "try before they buy."

The RESNA Technical Assistance Project provides technical assistance to the 56 state and territory assistive technology programs as authorized under the Assistive Technology Act of 1998 (P.L. 105-394). Readers can find out how to contact their state project by accessing the RESNA directory at http://www.resna.org/taproject/at/connections.html.

ABLEDATA, sponsored by the National Institute on Disability and Rehabilitation Research, is an on-line catalog of over 20,000 assistive devices manufactured by more than 2,000 companies. The URL is http://www.abledata.com.

CHAPTER FOUR

In God We Trust: A Brief Historical Review of Rehabilitation Practices

The past is a foreign country: they do things differently there.
— L.P. HARTLEY, THE GO-BETWEEN

The time in which Chuck, Brian, Jim, and Maggie live is like no other in U.S. history for persons with disabilities. Their constitutional right to life has come to be as much a guarantee of advances in technology, medicine and rehabilitation as it has human rights. They have the liberty to pursue all forms of happiness. Yet it is perhaps nowhere else more apparent than in the study of the history of the care and treatment of people with disabilities that there has been, over time, a cycle of waxing and waning in America's guarantees of freedom, equality, justice, and humanity.

It is important when discussing the current treatment of and attitudes toward persons with disabilities to realize that these do not occur in a vacuum — they are part of the complex and dynamic social, political, economic, and technological emphases at that particular point in time. To provide a context, this chapter provides highlights of the different "epochs" in our history to show how we have evolved over the past 200-plus years into a society that passes such legislation as the Americans with Disabilities Act, the Assistive Technology Act, and the Individuals with Disabilities Education Act.

EARLY INDUSTRIAL AMERICA

Man as a Machine

In pre-industrial America and during the early years of the Industrial Age, the majority of any given day was devoted to home maintenance and family and farm sustenance. As the Industrial Age began, household appliances and farming tools, though mechanically simple by today's standards, did much to help to reduce the workload. Early sewing machines, food grinders, and clothes wringers sparked as much affection for machines by those who worked in the home as the steam engine and cotton gin did for those who worked the land. Newly available mechanical devices were enthusiastically sought out by consumers and eagerly created by inventors.

More was becoming known about machines than about human anatomy. While more and more people were intimately exposed to the machine, few were privy to the inner workings of their own bodies. As medicine began to advance and Newtonian physics was being adopted as a world view, the analogy of the machine was often used to explain the mysteries of bodily structures, processes, and functions. Man came to be seen as composed of a set of mechanisms. This served both to mechanize humankind and to humanize machines.

As the Industrial Age progressed, machines came to be seen as viable replacements for weak or missing parts of the human anatomy. More sophisticated braces for arms, legs, and backs were forged. After the Civil War, prosthetic arms, hands, and legs were crafted that may appear crude by today's standards, but were actually vast technical improvements. Large numbers of manual wheelchairs, called "invalid rolling chairs," were produced as well.

In 1850, the U.S. population was 23 million. Twenty-five years later it had doubled. Railroads and tunnels linked persons and towns. Man's mastery over nature and machine appeared certain, and the young industrial society was based on the well-accepted premise that the machine and the factory represented the most advanced and efficient means to meet the burgeoning demand for goods. The factory, to be highly productive, had to be as well oiled as the machine. *Predictability, reliability, repeatability and synchronization* were considered crucial for maximum efficiency in mass production. These buzz words of the day shaped expectations for human performance and behavior as well — performance standards people like Jim or Maggie were hardly equipped to meet.

There were large numbers of people who were viewed as being unable to compete in our newly industrialized society without services to help restore function physically, mentally, emotionally, and socially. With the dawning of the Industrial Age and the movement of many families from farms to the cities, the response to people like Jim or Maggie was to ignore their needs and to exclude them from societal participation. Religious and other charitable organizations founded institutions, schools, and centers for persons with disabilities, but in the absence of national standards and guidelines, the quality of care varied widely. The gap between need and response to that need remained very wide.

20TH CENTURY AMERICA

Necessity — and wars — have been the mothers of invention for many things, including rehabilitation services. World War I was one of the many events to greatly change the treatment of individuals with disabilities from essentially *custodial* services to services emphasizing *rehabilitation*. With many soldiers returning without limbs, sight, or hearing, the Soldier's Rehabilitation Act was passed in 1918 to provide vocational retraining for veterans with disabilities. Soon thereafter, in the heat of debates and concerns about labor union demands for rehabilitation services for workers, the Vocational Rehabilitation Act of 1920 (Public Law 236) extended the same vocational benefits to civilians. This federal support was renewed annually until 1935, when rehabilitation programs achieved permanent status under legislative amendments to the Social Security Act. Rehabilitation services were initially provided only to those with physical disabilities.

In the mid-thirties and early forties, the debut of the antibiotic drugs, sulfa and penicillin, enabled medical professionals to halt many viral and postoperative infections. This, coupled with advances in casualty and trauma management learned on World War I battlefields, allowed significantly more people than ever before to survive major illnesses and injuries, although many with some form of permanent limitation or disability.

When American factories began to lose their workers to World War II, they hired women, minority workers, and individuals with disabilities to operate the machines and supply the war effort. Women, minority workers, and workers with disabilities found employment opportunities in wartime industries very attractive, and they did not want to relinquish their jobs to returning veterans when the war ended. Emerging from the war as a victorious and prosperous society with thousands of new jobs, postwar America could afford to be committed to both returning veterans and their replacement workers. In possession of the resources to become a more humane society, the United States entered a period of economic and social expansion.

Skyscrapers, suspension bridges, streamlined locomotives, airplanes, airports, automobiles, and an interstate network of concrete highways and service stations were all inspiring symbols of unprecedented personal and societal well-being. The appearance of television sets in middle-class homes in the early 1950s, the launch of Sputnik in 1957, the invention of the transistor, and the first Xerox copier in 1958 all signaled a new epoch in communication and the increasing role of electronics. The mass production and transportation of consumer goods heralded the growth of a consumer-oriented society. Machines had become the all-encompassing worldwide symbol of progress and prosperity.

The Change in Emphasis from PEOPLE to PERSON[1]

In the 20th century, our global focus was on tackling such mass population problems as the containment of contagious diseases and infection, sanitation, the construction of bridges and highways, and the implementation of public education. While education is in continuous need of updating and improvement, there is much work and repair needing to be done to our physical infrastructure, and there are disease processes still to be understood and controlled, we have made tremendous strides in conquering these massive, population-based, challenges. Today, we have a reasonably good service infrastructure and set of public policies and legislation internationally to protect and promote our health, safety, and education.

As I've attempted to depict in Figure 4-1 below, the 20th century focus was on people and their needs as a population. Often, each country had a fairly discrete population sharing a culture and language different from many other countries. The individuals comprising any given country's population were rarely the focus of attention, nor were products or devices uniquely shaped or crafted to fit individual needs and preferences. In the 20th century, it was common to have, say, one style of wheelchair prescribed for many people. Options and choices in wheelchairs and other assistive technologies, if they existed at all, certainly were not vast. And to better contain and control disease and disability, society decreed that people had to be treated and managed by healthcare providers. Services for people with disabilities and chronic health conditions, thus, came under the purview of medical professionals who, in keeping with their training, viewed disability against the normal curve of the state of the mass population's health and, thus, as a health problem which required treatment and cure.

In the beginning of the 21st century, less emphasis needed to be devoted to the service infrastructure and legislation and policy compared to the 20th century. Although refinements and advances will, and need to, occur there is now available time and energy to devote to the individualized needs of each *person*. No longer it is acceptable to have one wheelchair and expect that it will serve Jim, Bob and Juan equally. And Jim, Bob and Juan now have a legal right to have a voice in their choice of wheelchair. Thus, as depicted in Figure 4-1, the relative sizes of the circles representing areas of emphasis have changed over time.

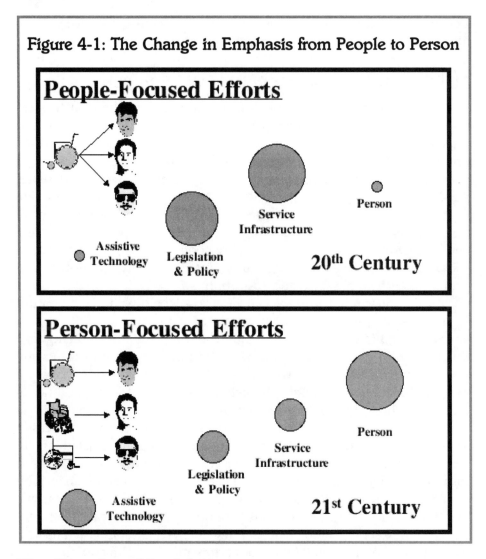

Figure 4-1: The Change in Emphasis from People to Person

Five Decades of Legislation

Persons, like Maggie, who were born with disabilities soon after the end of World War II had the benefit of the great advances made possible by increasingly sophisticated devices and dramatic changes in the concepts of rehabilitation fostered by treating the casualties of World War II. Not only were there more veterans who had survived the war, but thousands of them had no limbs, eyesight, hearing and so on. The enactment of the Vocational Rehabilitation Act Amendments of 1943 (Public Law 113) increased state vocational services and the funds needed to provide those services. Medical, surgical, and other physically restorative services were added to the concept of rehabilitation, and individuals with mental illness were added to the list of those eligible for rehabilitation services. Broadening eligibility for and types of services meant a dramatic increase in the number of persons with disabilities, and in those being served in rehabilitation facilities.

Rehabilitation mandates continued to expand through federal legislation. By the time Jim was born in 1957, the Department of Health, Education and Welfare was four years old, and Public Law 565, which authorized a nationwide system of training grants to increase the supply of rehabilitation personnel, had been in existence for three years. P.L. 565 also made grants available to help fund disability research and to test new approaches to rehabilitation. It provided the funds for the states to establish community rehabilitation programs. In 1954, another act provided badly needed construction monies for rehabilitation facilities. In 1965, Public Law 333 established behavioral disabilities and cultural and economic deprivation as conditions in need of rehabilitation services. Sheltered workshops, rehabilitation facilities, and self-help programs were encouraged or expanded.

The Sixties was a very socially conscious decade, with a conscious concern for social and racial equality. Ten years after the 1954 Supreme Court decision against segregated education in *Brown vs. the Board of Education of Topeka*, Kansas, Congress passed the Civil Rights Act (Title VI) of 1964 that ended segregation. Almost a decade later, civil rights were extended to individuals with disabilities under Section 504 of the Vocational Rehabilitation Amendments of 1973. The campaign for the signing of the 504 regulations was spearheaded by Dr. Frank Bowe as head of the American Coalition of Citizens with Disabilities (read Dr. Bowe's preface on pages vii–x). In the history of the disability rights movement, Section 504 represented a watershed in the coming together and solidarity of the disability community (Lathrop, 1997).

Section 504 gave individuals equal access to programs and services and mandated non-discrimination in federally supported education and employment programs. Segregated schools for children and adolescents with disabilities were starting to close. Many other legislative acts and governmental efforts also extended the rights of Americans with disabilities: The Rehabilitation Act Amendments of 1974 and 1978, the National Housing Act Amendments in 1975, the Education for All Handicapped Children Act of 1975 (Public Law 94-142 — popularly known as the "mainstreaming law"), the 1977 White House Conference on Handicapped Individuals, the Social Security Disability Amendments of 1980, and the designation of 1982-1992 as the international "Decade of Disabled Persons." Growth for rehabilitation resources and facilities had been legislated with the newly created Social and Rehabilitation Service in 1967, resulting in significantly broadened services for people with disabilities. Community rehabilitation programs and facilities sprang up by the hundreds, with widespread citizen support and involvement.

In the late 1960s, a group of students with disabilities formed an organization that evolved into the current Regional Center for Independent Living in Rochester, New York. In 1970 in Berkeley, California, Ed Roberts formed a group of students with disabilities called the "Rolling Quads." They moved out of the campus hospital (which was their dormitory) and into the community. Also in 1970, Judy Heumann started a similar group at Long Island University, called "Disabled in Action." These groups believed that the real issues facing people with disabilities were not medical, but attitudinal, political and economic — e.g., access to transportation, housing, personal assistance, and jobs. People with disabilities, they believed, should help other people with disabilities; those who have been through the experience know best how others might achieve independence. Working together, they asserted, people with disabilities could attain self-direction and manage their own programs. Thus the Independent Living Movement was born. The Rehabilitation Act Amendments of 1978 furthered this movement by fostering the establishment of Independent Living Centers throughout the U.S. It was one of these centers that Maggie was about to join as a new employee in 1986.

People riding in wheelchairs and modified vans, or walking city streets with guide dogs, burst out from behind closed doors and began to advocate for themselves and form coalitions and self-help organizations.[2] In the late 20th century, large numbers of people with disabilities were encountering one another daily throughout America. They started by actively working together in their own advocacy groups for a better quality of life through equal rights and accessibility. Before this time, advocacy group activities were run as charities by non-disabled individuals who would solicit contributions on behalf of persons with disabilities. The newer groups, run by individuals with disabilities, became heavily engaged in political lobbying and the development of public awareness programs. These efforts began to change the look of American cities and towns:

- Thousands of wheelchair ramps were built

- Notices in Braille were posted

- Traffic lights incorporated sounds to indicate *stop* and *walk*

- Handicapped parking spaces appeared

- Wheelchair-accessible toilets became available

- Telecommunication devices for the deaf became available as a supplement to regular audio telephone service

These efforts also had the cumulative effect of generating much optimism about the future quality of life for people with disabilities.

Rehabilitation was being redefined to mean not just the restoration of function, but also improving the quality of the lives of people with physical disabilities. Services were designed to assist individuals in returning to their communities so they could live independently and exercise as many free choices as possible. With institutionalization fast going out of favor, a tiered, community-based system was adopted offering foster family placements, group residences, and supervised apartments as residential options – particularly for those with developmental and psychiatric disabilities.

For persons with physical disabilities, assistive technologies became an area of increasing activity because they help persons live independently and enter the work force. Increases in the visibility of these devices impacted on community practices. For example, independent mobility by battery-powered wheelchair required accessible buildings and modified transportation systems.

Passage of the Technology-Related Assistance for Individuals with Disabilities Act in 1988 was closely followed in 1990 by the Americans with Disabilities Act (ADA) — which extended to individuals with physical and mental disabilities "reasonable accommodations" of their individual needs — and the Individuals with Disabilities Education Act (IDEA), which encouraged the consideration of assistive technologies in each relevant Individualized Education Plan. Legislation further accelerated the attention to the benefits of assistive devices. The Rehabilitation Act Amendments of 1992 facilitated the provision of technologies to eligible vocational rehabilitation consumers. In 1998, Congress amended the Rehabilitation Act to require Federal agencies to make their electronic and information technology accessible to people with disabilities. Section 508 was enacted to eliminate barriers in information technology, to make available new opportunities for people with disabilities, and to encourage development of technologies to achieve those goals. The law applies to all Federal agencies when they develop, procure, maintain, or use electronic and information technology. Under Section 508 (29 U.S.C. ' 794d), agencies must give employees and members of the public who have disabilities access to information that is comparable to the access available to those without disabilities.

The IDEA Amendments of 1997, the Assistive Technology Act of 1998 (P.L. 105-394) and President Bush's *New Freedom Initiative* further enhanced access to, and the availability of, assistive technologies.

Among the many goals of the *New Freedom Initiative* is significantly increased federal funding for low-interest loans so that more Americans with disabilities can purchase assistive technology. As a part of the New Freedom Initiative, the President issued Executive Order 13217, "Community-Based Alternatives for Individuals with Disabilities," on June 18, 2001. The Order called upon the federal government to assist states and localities to swiftly implement the decision of the United States Supreme Court in *Olmstead v. L.C.*, stating: "The United States is committed to community-based alternatives for individuals with disabilities and recognizes that such services advance the best interests of the United States."

A major victory for the funding of AT was achieved with Medicare coverage of Augmentative and Alternative Communication (AAC) devices. Effective in 2001, the Centers for Medicare & Medicaid Services (CMS) formally defines AAC devices as a Medicare benefit under the classification of durable medical equipment (DME). All Medicare beneficiaries are eligible for AAC device coverage, with the exception of skilled nursing facility (SNF) residents, as Title XVIII of the Social Security Act excludes coverage of DME within the SNF setting. In 2004, CMS launched *Operation Wheeler Dealer* to stop Medicare fraud in power wheelchair coverage and payment.

As much as assistive technologies themselves change over time, the legislation and policies affecting their availability also change. According to a 1990 National Health Interview Survey on Assistive Devices sponsored by the National Center for Heath Statistics and National Institute for Disability and Rehabilitation Research, 13.1 million or 5.3% of the total U.S. population in all age groups used assistive technology with 48.2% of devices paid for out of pocket compared to 34.0% paid by a third party. The remaining 17.9% were paid for by a combination of third party and out-of-pocket funds. In recent surveys, over fifteen million Americans with disabilities reported using assistive devices or technologies in recent surveys. (Carlson, Ehrlich, Berland & Bailey, 2001). It is likely many more individuals need and want AT but cannot afford to obtain it.

Figures 4-2 and 4-3 show the *interrelationships* among recent laws and the social/political climate in which they were enacted. For updates on legislation and government policies affecting persons with disabilities and assistive technology, please refer to Appendix C for links to web sites having the most current information.

Figure 4-2: Socio-Political Events

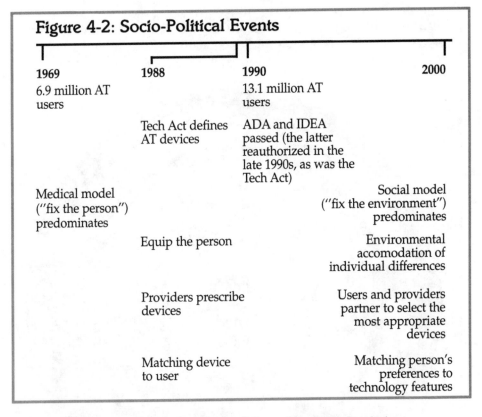

1969	1988	1990	2000
6.9 million AT users		13.1 million AT users	
	Tech Act defines AT devices	ADA and IDEA passed (the latter reauthorized in the late 1990s, as was the Tech Act)	
Medical model ("fix the person") predominates			Social model ("fix the environment") predominates
	Equip the person		Environmental accomodation of individual differences
	Providers prescribe devices		Users and providers partner to select the most appropriate devices
	Matching device to user		Matching person's preferences to technology features

Service Delivery: From Medical to Social Model

As we will explore further in the next chapter, professionals have tended to define goals achieved (e.g., independence) in terms of physical functioning whereas consumers more often equate independence with social and personal freedoms. A social model of rehabilitation views it essential to define the consumer's perspectives of the most desired outcomes.

Because we have largely succeeded in building our service infrastructure, and because we have the legislation and policies in place to protect our health, safety and rights, we can focus on the *person*. We have changed our focus from people with disabilities as belonging in the lower tail of the normal curve and requiring treatment and segregation, to the person with a disability and how obstacles to living in the middle (or higher) of the normal curve can be eliminated or minimized. We can refine AT products to conform to varied preferences and needs of individuals. It is precisely this availability of varied choice in technology features that has led to the existence of 20,000 different products.

Figure 4-3: Rings of Influence on the Degree of Match of Person and Assistive Technology (applies as well to Educational, Workplace, Healthcare and General Technologies)

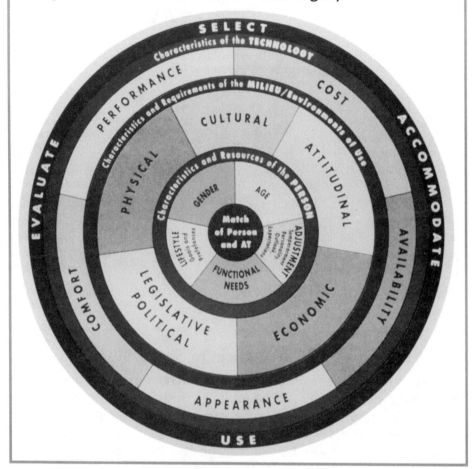

FROM THE INDUSTRIAL TO
THE INFORMATION AGE

Increasingly sophisticated machines and technology made it possible to mass-produce many of the major components of assistive devices. Together with the invention of the microprocessor in the mid-1970s, this made possible devices that were smaller, more portable and less expensive. Assistive devices thus became more affordable and more widely available. A physical limitation no longer prevented a person from participating in and contributing to society. Vocational rehabilitation counselors were knocking more frequently on employers' doors — and those doors were opening.

When personal computers became widely available by the mid- to late 1980s, electronic management of a broad range of tasks came within reach. Persons with severe physical disabilities were able to activate their powered wheelchairs with nothing more than a head nod, as Chuck does; those without intelligible speech, like Maggie, could finally express their thoughts by means of a computer's synthesized speech output. As machines and computers kept getting smaller and more portable, there seemed to be no constraints on dreams of complete freedom and unlimited opportunity.

The Glory Days Wane

By the mid-1980s, this rosy picture began fading. Government-sponsored programs cut back their services due to decreases in funding. Then, with the rise of managed care, rehabilitation units in hospitals found they had to push people out faster or lose money. The private rehabilitation sector, too, faced the need to trim programs. Those individuals who wanted or needed more long-term, intensive or specialized rehabilitation found themselves in the uncomfortable position of needing to establish their own fund-raising campaigns. Such individuals and their families began to air their appeals through the media and send out form letters soliciting funds. Families and individuals already emotionally taxed by the management of a disability now also felt degraded.

The hope of the day was that the quality of life for *all* persons with disabilities would vastly improve so they would have the *same opportunities* and resources as non-disabled persons. While we continue to empty the institutions, the moral equivalents of institutionalization and quarantine — stigma, isolation, and separation — continue to exist. Since older people with disabilities have not experienced the same opportunities for education and rehabilitation as younger individuals who have gone through the system more recently, it is not surprising that younger persons with disabilities are more frequently employed and better educated.

In 1800, farming characterized our economy. At the start of the 20th century, it was manufacturing. Now, at the start of the 21st century, it is electronics and telecommunications, information and knowledge — sectors where physical strength is not essential. No longer does a physical disability pose the barrier to employment it did during the past two centuries. However, the socioeconomic shift in focus from manufacturing to information management has especially disadvantaged individuals with cognitive, behavioral, and social deficits.

In education, employment, and elsewhere, the history of the United States shows that public support for assimilating people with disabilities into mainstream America has waxed and waned. Now, as we've entered the 21st century, persons with disabilities view their differences not so much as stigmatizing, but as markers of a different way of life, a culture. Yet, there is need to be cautious and to temper optimism. For example, the ADA faces continuous challenges, and the U.S. Supreme Court narrowed the definition of "disability" in 1999. As one person with a disability noted, "Our civil rights are like muscles — the more we exercise them, the more they'll develop, and what you don't use you'll lose" (Dragona, 1985, p. 35). This is as true today as when it was said in 1985. Shifts in national priorities and economics notwithstanding, civil liberties are fragile. Our experiences with mechanization and then computerization have made us a society accustomed to rapid changes and transitions — and their attendant uncertainty and frustration. From these changes may come an enhanced tolerance and respect for all individuals' human rights. In the meantime, who can help but be pleased by Brian's satisfaction with what he has accomplished in college — and on the ski slope? And can it be any wonder that Jim is awed by and grateful for the opportunity to walk out of his office building wearing a suit and carrying his work?

Footnotes Chapter 4

[1] This section originally appeared in: Scherer, M.J. (2002). The change in emphasis from people to person: introduction to the special issue on Assistive Technology. Disability & Rehabilitation, 24(1/2/3), 1-4.

[2] The oldest self-help organization in the United States is the National Association for the Deaf (NAD), founded in 1880.

CHAPTER FIVE

Rehabilitation Success: The Relativity of Theory

Doublethink means the power of holding two contradictory beliefs in one's mind simultaneously, and accepting both of them.

— GEORGE ORWELL, *1984*

CHRIS

I met Chris in the fall of 1985 at a day-long conference on computer devices for persons with physical disabilities. During the conference lunch, I was talking with the people at my table about various high-tech assistive devices and noticed, only peripherally, a tray being slid onto the table at the vacant spot to my right. This was followed by enough commotion of movement, clicking metal and audible huffs of exertion that my attention was drawn to the distracter.

A tiny woman in her early to mid-fifties, held up by metal crutches with cuffs around her forearms, loomed over me. She had a soft, kind face but one accompanied by an air of truculence. "Hi, sweetie. Mind if I sit here? My name is Chris Lofland. I'm OVR's[1] outback counselor. I say that because my office is in Greene County Hospital. I handle the spinal cord injured cases."

Her voice was strong, a little too loud, and though her words were friendly and warm, they came out crisp, pithy, sharp. Just a few years before, she had left a vocational rehabilitation job in New York City for one here and, in spite of her size and unsteadiness on her feet, retained about her that distinctive air of New York City toughness. As soon as she arrived, she had control over the table and never lost it.

Halfway through lunch she agreed to help me with my research. This bestowal of confidence encouraged another person at the table to do likewise.

We made an appointment to meet the next Friday at her office, the location of which she very precisely detailed to me. Unavoidably, however, I was running late that Friday.

While my mind was focused on meeting with Chris, I still couldn't help thinking, as I did every time I drove into the familiar parking lot at County Hospital, how very dreary and dismal the century-old place looks. While ringing the OVR doorbell at the foot of the ramp, I could recall the smell of urine, of human deterioration and decomposition there. Sometimes I swear I could take a sniff test long, long after I've left certain places and identify exactly when I was there, with whom, what I was doing, and how I felt about it.

I remembered the time I walked through an abandoned ward on the north side of this complex, looking for some old videotapes of interviews with patients and their families. The ward had been totally empty for five years, but the ward and its furnishings remained as they must have been on the last day of use, as though preserved as a memorial to hospital patients and practitioners otherwise long forgotten.

The beds were set three feet apart and lined both walls of the ward. One could easily imagine the people who had lain there over the past 100 years in pain and hopelessness. The stains on the mattresses, the smells that over many years had permeated the furniture and floors, the dismal atmosphere of death were going to hang in that stuffy, sunless, God-forsaken place forever.

The sudden opening of the OVR door startled me no less than Chris' friendly but brusque, "Hi, sweetie, come on in. You're late."

I sensed I shouldn't bother to explain the reasons for my tardiness. Sure enough, our first exchanges were to banter about youthful irresponsibility and mature experience. I knew I was getting a lecture frequently given to her clients.

Chris gave me a tour of the OVR suite, originally designed by the Occupational Therapy Department as a model apartment for retraining people to do homemaking tasks. In spite of Chris' hospitality and efforts to make it a homey and cheerful place, nothing could take away the dreariness of a suite of rooms in County Hospital.

We talked for a while in Chris' office — an average-sized room with an old wooden desk piled high with client folders. On the wall were photos of former clients, religious plaques, and Chris' framed certification. After twenty minutes or so, she suggested going into the kitchen area for coffee.

I knew from seeing and talking with her at the conference that Chris gets around using Lofstrand crutches, an electric scooter, and a specially equipped car. But this time, she eased herself up out of her desk chair, armed herself with a pair of wooden crutches, and made her way toward a wheelchair so old-fashioned in design and material that I commented on the use of such antiquities by a rehabilitation counselor in on the cutting-edge of high-tech assistive devices. She said the comfort and ease-of-use of her old devices couldn't be beat; "there's a lot to be said for old tried-and-true friends." Chris managed her transfer with enough awkwardness for me to offer aid, but she refused — and the next thing I knew she was seated and on her way towards the kitchen.

In the kitchen, over coffee, Chris made me feel like an old friend, a colleague and confidante. She told me she had contracted polio just before the age of two and had done most of her growing up in institutions. When speaking of her later work in New York City, she mentioned names like Howard Rusk[2] in the same casual manner she would refer to a member of her family.

Her first husband had also had polio. They adopted two daughters and had a happy marriage of twenty years before he died. Chris remarried, and her second husband (non-disabled) is now retired.

Chris had been awarded custody of her granddaughter (for a reason she didn't tell me) and was facing the child's return to her mother — a loss she dreaded. And she had just learned that her office was going to close at County Hospital and be rejoined with the main office downtown, which she also dreaded and was attempting to fight.

As for her job, she reported feeling torn many times between the "proper procedures" and doing what she feels would be most helpful for her clients.

> Too much help can be a disincentive to rehabilitation. They're better off if they have to fight some for what they want. But I can't be that hard. When they've shown they can use it, give it to them. Don't be stingy.

She seems to be genuinely concerned for her clients' quality of life, even though her primary focus on the job is their vocational rehabilitation. This she often finds frustrating.

> It often doesn't pay financially for them to go back to work. A good approach would be part-time work because they have to tack on getting-ready time and transportation. Too, their medical needs can be great. But this option is rarely there.

Then she leaned forward and, with a searching tone, added, "Why should we lose these people and these abilities?"

Being placed in frequent dilemmas has made Chris somewhat angry at the system, and she attempts to compensate by putting her humanity and genuine caring aside for an objective approach to rehabilitation. She has truly lived five decades of rehabilitation, as a consumer and then as a professional. Still, she encounters battles such as the most recent one involving her move from County Hospital back downtown.

She spoke not only of her clients but also of herself when she told me her perspective of *rehabilitation success.*

It's not just motivation, it takes a willingness on their part to work. They need to like a challenge... It's like 'I won this little battle,' and it builds you up.

Our coffee klatch over, we returned to her office where Chris proceeded to her file cabinets. Like a bibliophile showing off a prized collection of books, she lovingly touched each case folder as she commented on its thickness (a direct indication of her time and effort spent on the case) and gave a brief life-history of each person whose past and probable future lay patiently before our very eyes between the file folder covers. She selected a number of likely candidates for my research, then reached for the phone and called each of them to solicit their participation and cooperation with my project.

Chris's "tough-love" philosophy shone through clearly in the phone calls. With one client, she was direct and to the point, as though she was making a business arrangement. With another (Brian in Chapter One), she reassuringly coaxed, "Brian, your opinions are so very important... you are such a tremendous success, dear."

With one man who had become very obese and withdrawn, she turned to me as the phone was ringing and said, "This one may be tough." He answered. After a few moments of listening to him she disappointedly but sternly inquired, "What are you doing to yourself? Killing yourself, that's what! You big lug. C'mon, stop being so lazy. Your biggest problem is *you*, sweetie."

She did it. Chris got him to participate in my research. After she had hung up the phone, she turned to me with a worried look and said, "This guy needs a different approach."

After a few moments of thoughtful silence she added, "That was Butch. Let me know if you get any ideas for helping him, will you."

Always looking for a challenge. But it appears the system is starting to wear Chris down. Why should we lose these people and these abilities?

BUTCH, 1986

Because Chris had forewarned me about Butch's attitude, while driving to his house I was feeling quite apprehensive about meeting with him. It didn't help that it was eight o'clock on a dreary, dark March evening.

I drove up to a small Cape Cod-style house in the midst of a congested neighborhood. The house had a still, abandoned air about it even though I could see a couple of lights inside and could hear the faint sound of television. Yet everything seemed so quiet — there were no street noises, no dogs barking — and my knocks on the door sounded loud and aggressive.

After a wait of many minutes and some more knocking, no one came to the door. I got back in the car and deliberated about whether or not I should just leave, then returned to knocking on the door.

This time I heard movement inside and the door was opened by a middle-aged couple who looked at me as with as much apprehension as I was feeling inside. They were pleasant and polite, but without any delay escorted me upstairs to the long, dark entryway to Butch's annex, pointed me towards his door, and left.

Butch had converted the second floor of the house's detached garage into a large one-room recreation area to be his private domain. It was connected to the second floor of the main house by a long, gently sloped ramp/entryway. After ascending the ramp and coming to his door, I heard a husky, booming growl that set off just about every nerve in my body. "Came in the wrong way, didn't you! I told you to come the back way."

The voice quality was harsh, but the tone was one of gentle chiding. I opened the door.

Butch's appearance was as grizzly as his voice. A huge man (weighing about 460 pounds), Butch had a brown beard so long and thick that his entire face was covered except for his eyes. And those eyes. The right one was little more than a slit. His total appearance gave him the ability to call forth a foreboding and threatening persona at will. Apparently his overpowering frame and appearance did not provoke a visible reaction in me, and having thus given some impression of strength, Butch then let me see the gentle and sensitive man hidden inside. His very sadness and hopelessness immediately began to shrink his huge and threatening appearance to more ordinary and manageable proportions.

> I'll tell ya'. I had polio when I was 7. My left side was paralyzed. I fought and fought, and I came back from it... I'll be honest, that's one of the disheartening things about this. I fought so hard then, and came back, and now here I'm sittin'. There's no fightin' to come back.

Butch never married and, at the time of his accident, lived with his parents as he does now. His gross obesity is due to overeating and no exercise. It is painfully obvious that what was once muscle has become almost pure adipose. He had a heart attack when he was 26 years old, and at 38, it appears he's mercilessly teasing another. He says of his weight problem, however:

I weighed 200 pounds when I broke my neck... right now I weigh about 460... I just don't do nothin', don't do nothin' physical, nothin' mentally stressing or nothin.' I just sit here and enjoy it. The hell with it, that's the way I see it. No ambition at all, none. Went right down the tubes when I broke my neck. That's the God's honest truth. I'll eat right to the day I die. Have me another heart attack and get it over with. I'm just sittin' around waitin' now. The grim reaper's gonna toll one of these days. Does for everybody, so...

He paused and his affect suddenly mellowed. Then he said,

I enjoy eatin'. I'll be honest, I have very few things in the world I enjoy doin' and eatin's one of them.

His annex area, made possible by the financial help of no-fault insurance, has a wood-burning stove he uses in the winter to keep his place at about 75° to 80°. He needs it this warm because of his poor circulation. Yet he also needs to be cautious, since his body-temperature-regulating mechanism was affected by his spinal cord injury. He has an impaired ability to sweat below his level of injury and needs to protect himself from getting overheated.

His furnishings consist of a complete wet bar, a regulation-sized pool table, a wide-screen television, a short-wave radio ("I know as much as my police buddies do and sometimes before they do"), and some chairs and a couch for guests. He spends most of his time now watching television, and when he's feeling particularly inspired, he enjoys writing poetry. He then offered me "Coke on tap," saying that his place is the only private residence on the regular Coca-Cola delivery route.

There weren't many decorative furnishings, and a small artificial Christmas tree on the coffee table in March seemed to stand out. Given Christmas should be a rather painful time for him, since he received his injury in December, I wondered why he still had this Christmas tree on display. "Are you just late in putting it away or are you very early for next year?" (By this time, I was feeling relaxed enough to try a little chiding myself.)

"Oh, that's always there. My niece brought it to me in the hospital. Christmas is my favorite holiday."

Four years earlier, Butch had been driving home from work in his Corvette one late afternoon when an oncoming car without headlights struck him. His Christmas was spent that year in a state of semi-consciousness. He says he had a premonition that his accident would happen, but that he would be killed.

With a complete injury to his spine at the C7-8 level, Butch uses a power wheelchair to get around. It has a hydraulic lift that he took great pleasure in demonstrating. By pushing a single button, this huge man grew taller and taller until he towered above me, his head only one foot from the ceiling. He said this option is very useful for getting to those high, tough-to reach places, like top shelves in grocery stores. And didn't I agree that every grocery shopper would find this handy?

Butch has an elevator to take him up and down stairs, one that he and his brother designed and his brother and father built and installed. He only uses it to get to the dining room for meals and to go outside when the weather is good to feed the birds and squirrels that come into his yard.

He also has a fully equipped van that he no longer uses and a Jacuzzi that he can no longer fit into. This is a lot of expensive equipment to go unused, and I felt compelled to ask, "Is there anything that would make your van more appealing or useful to you?" Yet even as I asked the question, I could predict the tone of the response.

> I've lost my ambition to ride in vehicles. I've got about a million and a quarter miles under me and I've been about every place there is to be in this country, part of Mexico, and all over Canada and I've seen just about everything there is to see. Getting in that van and goin' down to the corner store... it just ain't worth that.

Then he talked about assistive devices in general and computers more specifically:

> They're a very poor replacement for what you used to have. And they don't even start to cover what you used to be able to do. And... I ain't no computer whiz. I don't ever want to be a computer whiz. I can't stand them; I hate to even look at the things. And all OVR wants to do now is push the computer.

Butch reported that he perceives himself as having adequate emotional, material, and physical support. He sees few people outside of family, but says he's always been a "loner." As for friends, he offered a rather glib response: "I've got no friends. Got rid of 'em all."

"Why? What do you mean, Butch?"

"Friends ain't friends, that's all."

While Butch is paralyzed from the underside of his forearms down, he has full voluntary control of his arms and hands. It was easy for him to grasp our glasses and work the Coke tap to fill them. He is the least severely involved of the spinal cord injured participants in my study, but compared to the other participants with spinal cord injuries, he received Chris' lowest rating on "adaptive behavior" (Brian had received her highest rating).

At the time of his accident, Butch was a driver for a garbage collection service. He says he loved his job.

> There's nowhere I could go and get paid what I was paid and enjoy it, or even do it the way I was doing it, so... You're sittin' here. You know it and you face it. Ain't no gettin' up and walkin' away, so... What can I say? I was used to it in the hospital. I didn't even wanna leave the ward. They had to pry me out of that place... [He choked up a little and then added] I was happy just stayin' there.

In the silence that followed, I thought about the traits ascribed to him in his psychological profile: *nervous, depressed, inhibited, quiet, hostile, impulsive,* and *indifferent*. These data, combined with what I'd been observing and hearing, made me ask about his attitude toward "getting on with life."

> **B:** I've got a real good *attitude*; it's my *outlook* that stinks.
> **M:** Well, how do you think you stack up against a 'rehabilitation success?'
> **B:** I haven't seen one success... I don't know what a success is, as far as sittin' in a chair. I don't know anybody that's a success sittin' in a chair unless they were that way before they broke their neck.
> **M:** How do you think, then, society defines it?
> **B:** Keep 'em out of sight, they're out of mind, period. If they don't have to look at ya' they don't have to think about ya.'
> As an example, there's this guy where my brother works. He's workin', but he's not a success. He's sittin' there gettin' $2 an hour less than everyone else in the place, the government's subsidizin' his work — and that's being a success? Wrong! No good.

I fished for his definition of his "life as a person with a disability," hoping I'd learn more about what makes him tick than I would from a more direct question.

> **B:** I wouldn't wish it on my worst enemy. I wouldn't wanna put any body in this position. There ain't nothin' worse than being stuck. There's nothin' you can do that's gonna change it physically and you know that right off the bat... And when you ain't got nothin' to fight with, then you lose your will. It makes me sick to think about [a $4-an-hour job]. Who needs it! I sit here with my television set; at least you know who you're talking to.
> **M:** Sounds like you're going to take your [life] and hide.

B: That's it. They ain't gonna get a chance at me. I don't wanna be their statistics or nothin.' I'm just sittin' here and enjoyin' it right to the day I die... whenever. Be it tomorrow, be it tonight.

M: Well, then, what would you say about the value of *accepting* a disability?

B: I'll look any son-of-a-bitch in the world straight in the face and say they never 'accept it.' There isn't a single person out there with a spinal cord injury that accepts what happened to them and doesn't wish they could get up and walk away from that chair and set fire to it.

I had asked Brian, too, if he had "accepted" his disability, and he had provided a very different response.

You have to accept it, you have to tolerate it. What else can you do? The way I overcome that disability, and the best way I've found, is not to think of it. Put your mind on something else or keep it busy enough where you don't think of it. Some people don't keep their minds occupied. When you think of that one thing all day, that's what's programmed in your mind. But again, that's your personality.

Chris sees Brian as a *rehabilitation* success and Butch as a *rehabilitation failure*. Both men, however, have accommodated themselves to lifestyles they believe to be the most tolerable way for them to live, at least for now. Who can say who's *well-adjusted* and who isn't? Who is and isn't a *rehabilitation success*?

Clearly, many of our cherished rehabilitation concepts are individual constructions.

THE DISABILITY EXPERIENCE

Chapter Four provided a historical perspective on the many changes that have occurred in the treatment and rehabilitation of individuals with disabilities. A more in-depth view of our present situation is essential for successfully addressing the needs and concerns of those persons who are living in the 21st century with a disability.

Each person who has spoken in these chapters has described his or her unique life experiences as a person with a disability, or what will be termed here the *Disability Experience*. The term is intended to refer to the "everyday experiences associated with [having a disability] as provided by individuals with disabilities in candid and intimate accounts" (Brightman, 1984). The individuals in this book have shown how the *Disability Experience* is both a personal and a social construction. While it is unique for each individual, it both shapes and is shaped by society's attitudes toward people with physical disabilities in general. The Disability Experience is, therefore, *an interactive one*. The discussion below illustrates this point.

Two Views

There can be critical distinctions between the perceptions held by people with acquired disabilities and those born with their disabilities. Individuals who have had whole new worlds opened for them through rehabilitation and technology, such as Jim and Maggie, see the value of assistive technologies differently from those who have had to leave the non-disabled world behind because of an injury, as Chuck and Butch did. Individuals with cerebral palsy able to speak for the first time because of communication devices can place a much higher value on that technology than the person who once had, but lost, the capacity to speak.

A 1983 article by Stoll and the one following it in *Disabled USA*, by Rosen, taken together, not only highlight the individuality of the *Disability Experience* and the variety of perceptions and responses surrounding it, but also show how this may be variously affected by the person's previous life experiences. Stoll (1983) emphasizes the role of laughter and humor in achieving a high quality of life. Stoll was born with cerebral palsy and was, therefore, socialized from birth as a person with a disability — her developmental history never included a time as a non-disabled person. Her perspective was like that of another person with cerebral palsy who said to me wryly during one of our interviews: "Having a disability is a tough job, but someone's got to do it!"

Rosen (1983) saw rehabilitation as a resocialization process for learning to become a "proper handicapped person":

> And so, in our defenseless state, without any psychological reserve at the ready, we began our first lessons in learning to be handicapped. (p. 7)

As Rosen's pre-injury view of people with disabilities was one of revulsion, he projected onto society and anticipated the same reaction to himself. Rosen, like Butch, had become "handicapped" by both society's beliefs about people with disabilities and his own personally and socially constructed perspective.[3]

It is true, however, that as part of a type of resocialization process, a person with a recent disability may be pressured to comply with rehabilitation practices that would be vigorously resisted by a non-disabled person. Professional intentions are to offer the best possible help, but they may unintentionally communicate the need for the consumer to become what Rosen calls a "proper handicapped person." While people are given therapy and training to minimize the importance of their disability in their lives, the concomitant message is given that the disability is so important as to require changes in the most basic elements of their lifestyles.

In Chapter One, Chuck provided an example of how well-intentioned professional objectives can become degrading and demoralizing. He underscored the problem this way:

> ...when you're in this condition, people say to you, "You've got to do it NOW." They don't look at it like they're looking at themselves, and saying, "I can put it off until later." ... I wasn't that organized before, so why should it change now? I know what has to be done and when it has to be done and that's what I work on. Your basic style doesn't change just because you're in a wheelchair...

The person with a disability can be placed in a no-win situation: To resist therapeutic advice is to risk unwanted physical consequences. To comply, however, may threaten one's self-esteem and need for self-determination.

PERCEPTIONS OF REHABILITATION SUCCESS

The Independent Living Movement focuses on self-directed choice and advocates the creation of opportunities for individuals to exercise as many free choices as possible. The working definition of *rehabilitation* used by most professionals is similar in its emphasis on the restoration of a person's physical, sensory, mental, emotional, social, vocational, and recreational capacities so the person can be as autonomous as possible and will be able to pursue an independent non-institutional lifestyle. To achieve this, the rehabilitation professional focuses on functional changes in the individual — through physical therapy, education, the provision of assistive devices, and so on — while simultaneously considering changes in the physical and social environment, such as the addition of a ramp to a house and the placement of the person into a special training program where there will be peer support. The ultimate outcome is intended to be improved well-being — both in terms of the actual physical conditions and the situations in which they live, but most importantly, as perceived by the persons themselves.

Rehabilitation success as a professional goal emphasizes the strengthening of physical, mental, social, educational and vocational capabilities and opportunities within the shortest possible time. This can mean helping a person *overcome* a functional limitation or *limiting its impact*.

Overcoming a functional limitation is the goal of physical rehabilitation (for example, regaining muscle control and strength so that the person can walk independently); limiting the impact of a disability on a person's life typically comes under the purview of psychosocial and vocational rehabilitation.

An "Ideal Client" Doesn't Need Rehabilitation

Professional definitions of rehabilitation success can seem very idealistic. Kaplan and Questad (1980) note that:

> A composite picture of an ideal client can be drawn from the studies reviewed in this paper. The ideal client would be a young, well-educated male with a slight physical disability who would be employed at the time of referral though not making too much money lest he be unmotivated. He would have a good self-concept, high self-esteem, independence, high motivation, specific goals for his rehabilitation, a stable work history, and would never have received public assistance. He would have a high degree of acceptance of disability, a high I.Q., and little need for emotional security. In short, the ideal client would probably not need much in the way of rehabilitation services (p. 167).

We are familiar with this view of rehabilitation success because it is the view presented in our newspapers, magazines and on television. It's okay to have a *little bit* of a disability. For anything more severe, the media focuses mainly on what people in this book have called the "super crips": the super-achieving persons with severe disabilities who outperform the majority of non-disabled people at some physical or mental task. It is also the case that media accounts can betray an attitude of discrimination and devaluation, although less in bold statements than in subtle, veiled putdowns that the author may not be aware of revealing.

Articles that try to portray a positive picture of persons with disabilities often end up being written in a patronizing, and thus offensive, style. Notice in the following example, the subtle — and not-so-subtle — put-downs in the first paragraph of an article on the Seventh International Summer Special Olympics:

> It was hot, the hot kind of hot Indiana hot weather that sends the family dog scooching under the pickup truck to enjoy the shade. But in South Bend, on the Notre Dame and St. Mary's College campuses, heroic athletes from 70 countries were running and jumping and laughing from the sheer joy of it all. No, these were not the Pan American Games, which were to start a few days later, downstate at Indianapolis. The com-

petitors there, everyone knew, would run faster and jump higher. But not happier; world happiness records were being set here at the Seventh International Summer Special Olympic Games (Skow, 1987).

The article appeared in the August 17, 1987 issue of *Time* magazine. Would this magazine have given an article on the Pan American Games a similar title — "Heroism, Hugs and Laughter" — or begin it with the same nursery-rhyme-style sentences?

And here is an example from a July 30, 2004 *Washington Post* article titled,"In Maryland, Disabled but Not Confined:"

> It is another sleepy Saturday evening at this Wheaton nursing home. Then the fiery woman in the red dress rolls off the MetroAccess bus in her electric wheelchair. She has a spiral notebook in her lap and passion in her voice. She's quadriplegic.
> She's Ellen Archie, 37. She used to live here. Now she's back, helping other people get out. "They can't stop you from having a life outside of here," Archie tells her old neighbors, who encircle her with their wheelchairs in the courtyard.

This article was actually very positive about Maryland providing waivers that allow nursing home residents ages 18 to 59 to opt for care in their own homes, provided they can acquire the home health services they need at the same price or less than it costs them to live in an institution. Yet, the writing style betrays an attitude of something akin to pity. Describing Ellen Archie as "fiery," having "passion", and being loyal and helpful to "her old neighbors" is not the kind of description she would likely give to, say, a non-disabled female attorney who volunteers in her spare time to advise nursing home residents of their rights.

Negative attitudes remain one of the biggest barriers to the full inclusion of people with disabilities in today's society. A 1991 Harris Poll on "Public Attitudes Toward People with Disabilities" revealed that people often expressed support of persons with disabilities as a general, abstract concept. However, when asked about specific situations, such as having a group home established in their neighborhood, they were considerably less supportive. In a 1998 Harris Poll, fewer than half (45%) of adults with disabilities say that people generally treat them as an equal after they learn they have a disability. The following excerpt from a 1992 article in the *New York Times* shows the public's apparent lack of sympathy for an individual with a disability who was innocently injured in an accident:

When a taxi jumped a curb in midtown Manhattan on Monday, two bystanders were struck and seriously injured. Since then, one victim has received four get-well cards. The second has received hundreds of cards; 300 to 400 people have called each day to ask about him, and well-wishers have contributed hundreds of dollars to insure that he receives good care.

The first victim is an elderly blind man. The second is his dog (Bennet, 1992).

Today, the same unconcerned attitudes toward persons with disabilities prevent an active commitment to their full and equal societal participation.

Consumer Motivation is Key

A cooperative consumer is said to exhibit a desire for independence and self-reliance while, at the same time, demonstrating a complete willingness to cooperate fully with rehabilitation therapists and other professionals. These apparently contradictory characteristics expected of a cooperative and "motivated" consumer can place the person in a no-win situation: Too much or the wrong kind of independence can be perceived as uncooperative; too much or the wrong kind of cooperation can be signs of passivity, depression, or dependence.

In the traditional medical model with a knowledge flow going in one direction only — from professional to consumer — individuals who place a premium on their independence, assertiveness, and self-direction may resent and confound attempts to help them. This may result in a no-win situation — a *state of stuck*.

Persistently uncooperative and unmotivated individuals have been portrayed as "demonstrating chronic, unmitigated disengagement from themselves, their family, goals, work and society" (Starkey, 1967). In addition, such individuals (like Butch) are described as angry and resistant to help. Their depression and hostility provoke rejection from their therapists and counselors, precisely the people who are there to help them. Thus, for the unmotivated consumer, a no-win situation can also exist.

In psychology, there are as many disagreements about the importance of motivation as there are theories to characterize and describe it. For example, Kaplan and Questad (1980) believe that the phrase "a well-motivated client" says more about congruence between consumer and counselor goals than anything about the consumer. Thus, the motivated consumer is one who likely resembles the therapist in many important ways, such as having similar background characteristics and placing the same value on education and work.

When a person with a disability has a different background or values from his or her therapist, the professional may believe the person will not succeed in rehabilitation and may unwittingly withhold resources and assistance, thus creating a "non-rehabilitated individual" as a *self-fulfilling prophecy*. When this occurs, the individual may indeed become stuck in a cycle of low motivation and poor functional gain. If the person is chronically depressed or passive, and feels he or she is "doomed to fail," he or she may be at risk for suicide and substance abuse.

Many Professionals and Consumers See "Success" Differently

Many rehabilitation professionals see the *Disability Experience* as fraught with obstacles and attitudinal barriers. Accordingly, they define "rehabilitation success" as coming as close as possible to non-disabled functioning. Rehabilitation professionals emphasize independence, maximizing individual potential, employment, and societal integration. They tend to judge individuals according to how well they meet this standard of success.

People with disabilities, however, say that "success" shouldn't require a comparison with non-disabled individuals. It's only meaningful to each individual according to what he or she can and wants to do. *Working* may represent success for one person, while *staying at home* may for another. They argue that when a rehabilitation system values only a narrow range of capabilities and goals, an individual's unique competencies and talents tend not to be cultivated.

Professionals and consumers often see things differently. But the views of individuals with disabilities also differ widely. Each person has his or her own preferences, perspectives, and expectations.

Ken, a 31-year-old man with a C5-6 spinal cord injury from a fall into a ravine behind his house when he was eighteen, has a bachelor's degree in social work and in 1986 conducted peer counseling sessions for an Independent Living Center. His adjustment to his injury was a long and painful process, not made any easier by the death of both parents a few years after his accident. As both a counselor and a person with a disability, he lives independently in an apartment after spending several years in his county's nursing home. About rehabilitation professionals emphasizing non-disabled functioning, he said:

This is very true. You go into rehabilitation and to them success is going out and getting a job. You can be just as much of a success by functioning at your highest capability — be it wherever, at work, college, or home. There are many rehabilitation successes in sheltered workshops. On the other hand, you can be working in a competitive job and doing a good job, but if you're not working at your full capabilities, then you're not a success. In the public's eye, and in those of many rehabilitation professionals, a rehabilitation success is making $50,000 a year, living in a big house and having three kids. This is the model of rehabilitation held up to us. It does a lot of harm to individuals' self-image, and it also encourages society to keep holding this model up. Everyone loses.

Chris and Butch provide just two examples of how a counselor's and a consumer's perceptions of "success" can differ. Even when a rehabilitation professional and consumer may seem to agree on the surface, a closer look into their definitions usually reveals the professional's focus on minimizing physical limitations.

A rehabilitation engineer, for example, defined *rehabilitation* success as being limited to the work done by the seating clinic:

If through the work we've done we have increased the person's independence, or [created] a safer and healthier situation (for example, we've provided a seating system that avoids pressure problems), that is what I consider a success.

A man with a spinal cord injury, however, defined *rehabilitation* success more broadly in terms of *psychological well-being* and as being more related to the standards of particular individuals.

A rehabilitation success is any way you can resume a 'normal' life, no matter if for you a normal life is staying at home. Just as long as you can keep on going with a decent frame of mind. Being successful is just being able to go on living. Being successful is living the way you want to live. You can be successful sometimes and unsuccessful others. It's not an absolute. There's probably as many definitions as the people you're talking to. Part of that is just personality... [and frame of reference].

As noted earlier, even when only comparing the perspectives held by people with similar disabilities, it is clear that two individuals (like Brian and Butch) can have two very different views of "success."

For the most part, however, individuals with physical disabilities agree that the meaning of the term *rehabilitation success*, like the *Disability Experience*, depends on individual capabilities, preferences, and experiences. Most individuals see themselves as a success in their own way, and tend to speak in terms of doing what they themselves want to do and achieving a level of independence that is personally satisfying. They recognize and accept that physical rehabilitation is not physical restoration. They seem aware of the distinction between acceptance of physical limitations and a focus on negative aspects of the disability and limitations.

Some examples of the views of *rehabilitation success* held by people with cerebral palsy or spinal cord injuries follow. Their definitions are more similar than they are diverse, and they highlight many of the same elements: personal contentment and satisfaction.

CHUCK:
Anybody is successful if they are home, and that's where they want to be, and doing okay. As long as they're happy and content with where they are. My idea of success hasn't changed, whether I'm in a wheelchair or not.... If I decided right now that I didn't want to pursue the computer and wanted to do something else, regardless of what it was, and never left home and was happy, then that would be a success. To me, being unsuccessful is being stuck in a situation you can change and you don't do it, and you're not happy with your present situation.

MAGGIE:
People with enough faith in themselves.

D.E. (cerebral palsy):
Being as independent as your disability allows. Everybody is a success in his or her own way.

S.T. (spinal cord injury):
Being able to live independently and doing what you want to do as opposed to withdrawing from the world.

T.E. (cerebral palsy):
I'm a success because I'm not in an institution. A good mental state is everything. I'm making my own decisions, I got married, I'm living as full a life as I can.

The different perceptions of rehabilitation success held by people with disabilities and the professionals who work with them may or may not influence the rehabilitation relationship and the resulting services provided. However, if rehabilitation professionals and engineers attend primarily to a functional limitation, and do not consider the individual's emotional and social situation and concerns, the *person* they are striving to help may feel secondary to the disability. Thus, it just may be that the most motivated consumers are those involved in a situation where a particular counselor and consumer have established a rapport and share the same perceptions of rehabilitation success.

Footnotes Chapter 5

[1] OVR stands for "Office of Vocational Rehabilitation." While the name may change from state to state, OVR offices throughout the U.S. are federally mandated to help people with disabilities prepare for and retain jobs. This involves arranging for medical, psychological, and vocational evaluations and providing guidance and counseling, job training, job seeking skills, work adjustment, and job placement services. Many Independent Living Centers, VR offices and Client Assistance Programs in the U.S. are funded through a single state budget.

[2] Howard Rusk, M.D. (1901-1989) is known as the "father of rehabilitation medicine," establishing the field internationally as an important new medical specialty. New York University Medical Center's Howard A. Rusk Institute of Rehabilitation Medicine is named in his honor. At the heart of Dr. Rusk's approach to rehabilitation medicine is the concept that it should focus on the whole person (Perkes, 1995).

[3] Another excellent example of this phenomenon is discussed in Scott's (1969) book, *The Making of Blind Men: A Study of Adult Socialization*. Scott's study reveals ways in which behaviors commonly associated with blindness result more from learned social roles than from anything to do with the loss of sight.

CHAPTER SIX

Struggles and Strivings

What reinforcement we may gain from hope;
If not, what resolution from despair
— JOHN MILTON

Most professionals tend to believe that rehabilitation success requires a state of mind, an attitude that motivates individuals to work hard on their rehabilitation plans. They focus on functional independence, increased capabilities, and the ability to overcome environmental barriers. As Chris said when asked to comment about this,

> I agree. Rehabilitation professionals definitely see it that way. But the law says that we must have the goal of employment or independent living in the community.

Such a perspective on the part of professionals is fostered by a rehabilitation system that emphasizes the achievement of societal valued outcomes such as job placement and independent functioning. Individuals with disabilities, however, favor an overarching emphasis on quality of life — one that they individually construct and that extends beyond functional gains.

Assistive technologies are seen as valuable enablers of such accomplishments as employment and independent living. Accordingly, when professionals are asked to list the major advantages of assistive technologies, they mention improved functioning, increased capabilities, enhanced independence and less often mention quality of life.

When rating users' functional capacities for this study, professionals gave perfect "adaptive behavior" ratings to device users, regardless of disability type. Device users with either spinal cord injuries or cerebral palsy rated themselves on the Personal Capacities Questionnaire as exhibiting more "adaptive behaviors" than did people not using devices. Thus, all users of devices were seen by both themselves and their counselors as exhibiting more socially and personally adaptive behaviors than non-users.

A focus on the need for individuals to enhance their functional capabilities and to adapt themselves to their environments reflects the traditional *individual deficit modification* model of rehabilitation, commonly referred to as the *medical model*. This model stresses the importance of changes in the consumer. A high value on assistive technologies is consistent with this perspective. *Environmental deficit modification* focuses on ways to alter the environment so as to facilitate the integration of people with functional limitations into society. It is the philosophy behind such legislation as the Americans with Disabilities Act, and is representative of a *social model* of rehabilitation that emphasizes an environment where "everyone fits" and the need for individualized adaptations and accommodations is reduced

Writing for a special issue of *Computer* magazine, an engineer expressed the view that "handicapping conditions" occur when a mismatch exists between an individual and that person's environment. The mismatch can be corrected in one of two ways: the individual's capabilities can be enhanced, or the environment can be modified. He went on to say,

> In a world where human beings and the machines they command have the power to control the quality of life, handicapping can only be the result of failure to properly apply technology or the neglect of its development (Rahimi, 1981).

Two other engineers also see assistive technologies and environmental modifications as the primary solutions to the functional limitations of a physical disability:

> There are two models or approaches from which to work: (a) modify the world or (b) equip the individual.

> There is nothing wrong with disabled people that the proper environment can't fix... Technology can solve anything... the problem is to get people to use the devices.

Consistent with these statements is the belief that a person's quality of life will be high once he or she is enabled to walk (or talk, see, hear) and once he or she is gainfully employed. When coupled with an attitude of "knowing what is best" for the person with a disability, the tendency for technology specialists is to view assistive technology as the crucial — and sometimes the only — factor needed for successful rehabilitation and, therefore, quality of life. Today, the prevailing perspective is that *both* environmental modification and "equipping the individual" are necessary.

> Rehabilitation professionals must know assistive technologies, know the consumer, and involve the consumer. While rehabilitation professionals and consumers often share the same goals, professionals have not traditionally involved the consumer as an equal partner in the rehabilitation process.

The economic costs of individual rehabilitation and environmental deficit modification may be high, but society's emotional investment is low. So, too, is society's investment in the psychosocial needs of individuals with disabilities. We are currently making widespread environmental accommodations and are creating more and better technologies that minimize the *functional* impact of a disability, yet we often fail to provide the more intangible but essential opportunities for assimilation. While accessibility and enhanced functioning are important goals, many persons with disabilities believe more crucial are an individual's basic needs for security, autonomy, affiliation, accomplishment, intimacy, and identity. As outlined by Norris Hansell (1974) in his discussion of people's essential attachments, individuals need to feel connected to the world in which they live — connected to other persons, connected to a social role — to feel that they matter and that their lives are meaningful. *That* is quality of life.

AN ALTERNATIVE PERSPECTIVE: KEN, 1988

Rehabilitation professionals and engineers strive to minimize disabilities and remove the environmental barriers faced by persons with disabilities. However, people with disabilities desire a more *person-centered* perspective. A professional who also has a disability illustrates this concept.

Ken

Ken, first discussed in Chapter Five, is a social worker with a C5-6 level spinal cord injury from a fall. He uses a power wheelchair, modified van, and a variety of low-tech assistive devices. He is so tall that the roof on his van had to be raised to accommodate his height when sitting in his power chair. His brown hair is fairly long, and he wears wire-rimmed glasses.

In 1988, Ken was a peer counselor for an Independent Living Center. It is easy to see why he would choose social work for his career. His facial features and expression are gentle and he has a soft-spoken, calm and kind demeanor. His responses are thoughtful, insightful, and sincere. He comes across as someone who could take charge, get the job done, but in a quiet, low-key manner. Everything about Ken says he is truly caring and sincere, but a sadness, a resignation, in his tone betrays the fact that he became who he is in a rather arduous way.

As a peer counselor working for an Independent Living Center, Ken is very active in his community in advocating civil rights for persons with disabilities. His major concern at the time of this interview was increased access to buildings and public transportation. Yet, the first topic he brought up during our interview was a new kind of power wheelchair that can go up and down stairs. He was very intrigued by this wheelchair and hoped that he might be able to have one in the near future. I asked him, "Do you think that's where they should be spending their research dollars, in equipping individuals so that they can go in any building? Or should they be making buildings accessible regardless of the person's means of mobility?" He responded as follows:

> Ideally, you make the building accessible. If you can do that, then each person does not have to have a different adaptation to get into the buildings. Philosophically, if the building is accessible then the person will feel more comfortable going into it — as if they're accepted into the building. If you have to adapt yourself to go into a building, it's like they're saying, "Well, okay, we really don't want you here, but if you can figure out a way to get in, we'll allow you to come in."

We continued to talk about the need for improved assistive technologies, access to buildings and the price tag of accessibility. Ken's own words summarize this discussion well:

> So, instead of going for the real luxuries, as far as wheelchairs that can go up and down stairs, you first need to cover the basics. It doesn't matter if you can go up and down stairs if you're starving to death because you are alone and you can't get the food to your mouth. First put the money into the necessities of life.

In contrast to the disability-centered viewpoint traditionally held by rehabilitation professionals, the *person-centered perspective* focuses on attitudinal and psychosocial changes that enable people with disabilities to participate more effectively in mainstream society. The goal is to create the best personal, social, and environmental climate for individuals with disabilities to achieve their needs for security, autonomy, affiliation, accomplishment, intimacy, and identity within the larger society. As Ken said, accessibility carries with it a message of inclusion.

INDEPENDENT LIVING PROGRAMS: PEOPLE FIRST

Ken is just one of thousands of individuals with disabilities who have adopted an Independent Living (IL) philosophy. The Independent Living Movement, discussed briefly in Chapter Four, was started by a group of persons with disabilities who were determined to exercise choice and maximize opportunity and individual autonomy. By 1978, more and more persons with disabilities had moved into mainstream America, and both the need and the desire for institutional care were greatly diminished. The 1978 Amendments to the Rehabilitation Act of 1973 (P.L. 93-112) and the Rehabilitation Comprehensive Services and Developmental Disabilities Amendments of 1978 (P.L. 95-603) provided federal funds to states for the establishment of Independent Living services. Today, there are four core services that federally funded independent living centers must provide (Smith, Frieden, & Richards, 1995):

1. Information and referral.

2. Peer counseling.

3. Independent living skills training.

4. Individual and systems advocacy.

Centers may also provide such services as housing assistance, architectural and communication barrier consultation, personal counseling that is non-clinical and short term in nature, assistance in acquiring and maintaining appropriate benefits and entitlements, and help in securing, learning how to use, repair, and maintain equipment.

It may sound like a contradiction in terms, but *Independent Living* can focus as much on interdependence as it does on independence. In addition to peer assistance, persons with disabilities acknowledge the important role of educators and rehabilitation professionals in their attainment of an autonomous lifestyle. A supportive family is also important — especially when family members provide care and act as personal assistants.

Assistance is Often the Key to Independence

Assistance from others *can* enhance a person's autonomy. To work or attend school, approximately 20% of persons with disabilities require help in such daily self-care activities as bathing, dressing, and feeding. Family members (parents, siblings, spouse) are the providers of such assistance for over 80% of those persons who require it. According to Nosek (1990), other options for personal assistance include:

a) paid assistants, either full- or part-time;

b) assistance arranged through a "barter system" where room and board, for example, are exchanged for assistance;

c) a shared assistant between roommates or another person with a disability who lives nearby.

Consumers believe they have more dignity and can exercise more control with paid assistants, but often do not have the funds for such assistance. Thus, there is often a trade-off between low- or no-cost family-provided assistance and other, more costly arrangements.

Each person needs to find his or her own balance of independence, interdependence, and dependence. As paradoxical as it may sound, assistance from others can enhance a person's independence.

Nosek (1990, p. 3) outlines three levels of need for personal assistance:

a) *Extensive*, for persons who could not perform survival functions under any circumstances. [Chuck and Maggie fall into this category.]

b) *Moderate*, for persons who could perform functions autonomously in emergency situations but require assistance to manage with a reasonable degree of efficiency. [Brian and Ken require this level of assistance.]

c) *Minimal*, for persons who could perform functions autonomously but choose to use assistance to conserve energy and/or time, or to minimize discomfort or damage to weakened muscles. [Butch and Jim are examples of people needing minimal assistance.]

How individuals achieve independence while managing their needs for personal assistance is highly individualized, as the following examples illustrate.

Brian, 1988

In June, 1987, Brian graduated from college and then drove his van coast-to-coast (camping all the way) to live in Berkeley, California. He came home for a short visit the following summer.

> Berkeley is great. I definitely have learned a lot since I left. And that was the whole purpose behind leaving; to learn more and to experience more and to live a fuller life. Not that I wasn't living a full life here, but I knew

there was more of a life out there. Here, when you're out in the country and there's snow everywhere, you're kind of caught up in your own little space.

It's quite a mind-blowing thing because you have so much freedom, so much independence around there. I mean, there's so many people that are in chairs and so much stimulation because there are so many people around. And there's a lot of people I've met that have been attendants — they've recently jumped into the area and needed some money. They needed a job real fast and this was a way for them to help somebody else and get some money at the same time. It's human relations and a great way to meet people.

Right now my big interest is in recreation. That's where I met Barb [his current girlfriend, who accompanied him on this trip home]. It's a great way of getting out in the community and meeting people. Once you get out into the outdoors, it makes... it improves your self-esteem.

I've been out in California a year now and feeling as independent as I can. I've been feeling out my values and looking at what's going to please me, what's going to make me happy in life. I've really taken this year off from work to do that. Now I think I don't want engineering, but something working with people, where I feel I'm benefiting society. Just before I left, my new OVR counselor called and said, "How'd you like a teaching position?" And I was just like, "Whew, that sounds great." It would be at a college helping teach math to students with learning disabilities. And I love math. It's half-time, so I wouldn't be losing many of my benefits — which is very important when you think about making any sort of big money. Hey, if I got an engineering job, all my benefits would be cut off! I'd rather have a part-time job, keep a lot of my benefits, and have a lot of free time to do things outdoors like kayaking, sailing and rafting. But working and making money is also important, and I can satisfy my needs to help by teaching.

When Brian lived at home he relied on his family for some of his personal care needs. I was curious if he now had a personal assistant.

Through the months I've had a series of roommates. Right now I have a guy from Boulder who helps me with showers, and getting up. I had a girl roommate for three months and she helped me out, too, and we got pretty close. Yet, those things can get too close and, it's like a big slice down the middle. Now that she's gone we've gotten real close again.

Personal assistance needs to focus more on issues of privacy and dignity.

I really don't need that much personal assistance. And the care that I need, I just ask for it in the morning and at night; the rest of the time I take care of my own apartment and meals.

But I do want that humanistic part. Without people, I wouldn't be where I am now. When I was in the hospital right after my accident, if I didn't have my family and friends coming up and seeing me, encouraging me... I learned off myself talking with other people and it's just evolved. That's why I don't think robotics are the answer for people with disabilities. For example, one of my favorite times was when someone was feeding me. We'd get some good interactions going. You can't do that with a robotic device. It's like... to have your needs met by a robotic device is like saying you're subhuman. But to have someone assist you, to have that conversation, to get to know and live with somebody, it's affirming your value as a human being. It's really important when you can hook up and be just like anybody else and you have human needs that need to be met and the other person can get the same fulfillment out of it. My roommate now gets more out of helping me than I get out of having help. It's giving him a lot of satisfaction. And better understanding.

And so, yeah, it's been a year and I've come back and I've seen everyone. And I said, "Look, you guys, it's been a year. How have you expanded in a year? This is how I've done it." I've learned a lot of things. But now it's time to go back there and start a new direction.

Brian illustrates several of the important dilemmas that persons with disabilities face. One is the trade-off between a full-time job and the loss of benefits when one's income exceeds the limits set by public sources of support. Another is the management of intimacy and dignity in the face of dependency. The third is achieving a balance between independence and interdependence.

Technologies are being developed to replace the need for expensive, intrusive, often unreliable assistance from other persons. But, as Brian expressed, care cannot be reduced to a technical task. It involves human judgment and understanding. To try to replace more and more interpersonal elements with technical ones can disconnect the individual from contact with caring, supportive persons.

Similarly, we just do not know all of what is involved when human parts and functions are increasingly replaced by technological substitutes. Zola (1984) indicated that it is a mixed blessing. The physiological body rejects transplants and skin grafts that it feels are alien to it. So, too, the psychosocial person rejects parts that he or she feels are alien. The more dependent the person feels he or she is on technology for life support and maintenance, and the more internally attached and dependent on machines the person becomes, the less the person's emotional needs are being met or addressed.

The best assistance is a blend of caring and support with task accomplishment. Technologies can help with the latter, but not the former.

Jim, 1988

Jim's pride in "walking out of the building with a suit on" has given him the desire to be more like his colleagues at work in all other ways. Because his capabilities were so restricted or "hidden" until his early twenties, his newfound freedom has created a desire to cast off both dependency and interdependency in all areas of his life. In 1986, Jim explained:

I like to have a party once a year for the people I work with. It's amazing how differently they treat me afterwards when they've seen me on my own time. "My goodness, Jim, you really can do this all by yourself!" They become more relaxed and open. We were just talking a few minutes ago and it's funny, I realized I'm more comfortable around normal people and I think I'm more like normal than handicapped people.

I have a friend with CP, Nancy. After that party I had, she and I went to a CP group and I was uncomfortable and miserable. I'm used to people who do a lot of thinking and talking about work. I couldn't relate to these people because most of them are living at home or working in sheltered workshops.

Nancy reminds me so much of me before my education and rehabilitation. And I was so wrapped up in her... she doesn't want to work — she dropped out of college because they did not let her study what she wanted to and she thought she would pay them back by quitting college. She thinks about her mother dying, and she wants to die with her mother because nobody will take care of her. I am more relaxed at work and am more comfortable with normal people. But I was ready to give up work and go with her because I wouldn't have to worry about bills and keeping house. But I got to thinking, "This is okay, but Monday morning will come and I'm going to work. If I marry her I lose doing things with my friends at work." I like Nancy, and I think she likes me, but we're often at one another's throat. Even my mother said, "It'll never work," and I was surprised because she always said, "Marry a handicapped girl." I want to be like able-bodied people but I don't think my parents have caught up with this yet.

I have too many friends whose parents despise me to death because I'm so outgoing and I don't let my handicap stop me. I'm a threat to their need to martyr themselves.

Many of today's adults with cerebral palsy have not led emotionally, socially, and cognitively enriched lives. Since early childhood they were not given many opportunities for socialization activities, such as talking with others and sharing ideas and experiences, especially if their speech and communication skills were poor. Typically they have not had the opportunity to use these types of interactions to help them establish a firm identity. Often, one effect of assistive devices can be to thrust them unprepared into a very different world, and this can produce tremendous culture shock. Thus, even though trained in accounting, the opportunities presented to Jim until recently prepared him more for a life of dependency than for one as a successful accountant. The more subtle aspects of his career status, such as managing his own finances, were challenging — as he described in 1988:

> The government handouts did good for me. They allowed me to get an education and gave me everything I need but I really did not learn the true value of money until... and am still learning it... when I needed something the money was always there. I didn't understand that it could stop or run out someday. So when I started working I took a cut in money and it took me five years to catch up. Of course, people need the money and the help. But at the same time they need to realize that it isn't always going to be there. And at first, I lived from payday to payday. But I'm learning, and I saved and now I have my own condo. Getting it is definitely not the same as earning it.

Jim's family, always supportive of him, apparently was not prepared for his degree of independence and in some respects continues to treat him as irresponsible. Jim very much resents this:

> My family was always supportive of my independence and allowing me to try things out but lately, every time I go back... I get mad at my dad so much! He would rather put down somebody in the family than quarrel or disagree with the person he's really angry with. Now every time we get together with the family he has to get on my case about something, like finances. Then they wonder why I get into a bad mood! I said, "Dad, can you get a hold of four thousand dollars right now?" And he said, "No." "Then why are you bothering me?" Actually, I couldn't either, but he didn't know that.

Jim's "teenage rebellion" is a healthy one, albeit delayed until his thirties. Some individuals with either congenital or acquired disabilities, particularly those whose family did everything for them, can exhibit learned helplessness: because they are dependent, they feel powerless, and they conclude they are unable to overcome their limitations and their dependency. Such persons may settle into a passive-dependent lifestyle, doing only those things that invariably reinforce their view of themselves as "disabled." Ken articulated this as follows:

> Sometimes you get lost between non-disabled and disabled thinking. I know myself, I side with the non-disabled more. Assistive devices can help improve integration with the non-disabled. If you don't integrate, you fall in more with being disabled and may have more of an institution-alized attitude.
>
> People who don't use assistive devices tend to rely on other people and tend to stick with people the same as themselves — who don't use devices either. That's what I mean by an institutionalized mind set. They also tend to believe they don't have control over their quality of life and that community integration is unattainable. For example, alcoholics tend to stay with other alcoholics because they have the same framework. If the people you're with don't keep up with your attitudes, you change to a different group. If you don't want to change groups, then don't change your attitudes.

Jim discussed people who lead passive-dependent, "institutionalized" lifestyles when he talked earlier about his friend Nancy and the members of the CP group he observed:

> I'm used to people who do a lot of thinking and talking about work. I couldn't relate to these people because most of them are living at home or working in sheltered workshops.

Jim's therapist discussed this from her perspective:

> Institutionalized people had everything done for them — their meals cooked, their beds made — and now they fight independence all the way because they lost that critical point where every kid wants to move out of the nest and be on their own. The more severe the disability, the more true this is because people really cannot do many things for themselves. You want people to keep believing they have some control and that something new and exciting can still happen to them. Institutions can sap people of that. Families, too — especially if they martyred themselves and ended up stifling the child and themselves.

Jim, himself, makes a strong distinction between people who are and are not self-sufficient and seems to have internalized the view that those working in sheltered workshops are inferior. Since he aspires to be a "normal person," he avoids others with cerebral palsy, saying he is more comfortable around those who are "normal" and share more of his interests. He has yet to grasp, however, many of the more subtle aspects of his career status and desired lifestyle, like the way he dresses for work, manages his finances, and handles challenges from his father. When corrected or challenged, he feels victimized.

The Desirability of Being Both Person - and Disability-Centered

Those who look beyond an individual's disability and believe it is ultimately more important and cost-effective to enhance a person's quality of life, not merely to restore capability, are being *person-centered*. Individuals with this more comprehensive perspective see the environment as presenting barriers and challenges, but also as stimulating and offering opportunities for accomplishment. Assistive technologies must pass the acid test of fostering independence and autonomy and contributing to a positive identity, enhanced self-esteem, and improved quality of life as defined by that particular person.

Being person-centered means looking beyond environmental accommodations and individual functional capabilities to the achievement of a higher quality of life. Assistive technologies can be important enablers in achieving a more satisfying quality of life when they address a person's emotional and social needs and preferences.

QUALITY OF LIFE[1]

In 1983, Elizabeth Bouvia made headlines. At age 26, she had lived most of her life "completely disabled by cerebral palsy." With a clear mind but a body in tremendous pain (she also had arthritis), she asked a hospital to permit her to starve herself to death, saying, "You can only fight so long. It's more of a struggle to live than to die."

Elizabeth made the news, not so much because of her desire to end her life, but because of the ethics involved in her efforts to die assisted by the medical profession. The sentiments Ms. Bouvia expressed are not uncommon among individuals with severe disabilities who are in constant pain and who feel they have a poor quality of life. For example, Maynard and Muth (1987) reported the case of a man with a severe spinal cord injury who made the decision to end his life, and did so. In a case presentation for the American Paraplegia Society, an ethically, clinically and legally sound process for treatment withdrawal was discussed (Butt, 2004). While in 2004 some individuals with severe disabilities may choose this option, there are many other individuals who, when presented with the means to function relatively independently and achieve valued goals, change their minds (as Elizabeth Bouvia did) and go on to lead long and personally satisfying lives. What may appear to be a bleak existence one day can be changed to a life of well-being and fulfillment — in spite of challenges and obstacles.

Today, physicians and other health care providers are paying more attention to "the life the consumer will have after you save his life" (Scofield, 1999). Yet current perspectives and definitions of *quality of life* are fraught with a vagueness that is compounded by the fact that technologists and rehabilitation professionals often have a tendency to make value assumptions about the needs of people with disabilities. As noted in Chapter Five, such assumptions often say much more about professional attitudes and beliefs than about the people they are trying to help. For example, Evans and his colleagues (1985) compared kidney transplant and dialysis patients on their self-reported quality of life. Many of the hemodialysis patients expressed life satisfaction even though they endured under very trying circumstances. To them, dialysis was an opportunity offering life itself. While the quality of life for people with end-stage renal disease may appear bleak by objective measures or professional viewpoints, the individuals' own subjective self-reports can be quite positive. The authors appropriately note that such incongruity underscores the need to consider quality of life as a highly individualized state that varies over time, and even day-to-day, rather than as a stable trait. A crucial point, then, is that people can "adapt to very adverse life circumstances, expressing satisfaction with their lives" (Evans et al., p. 58). Whiteneck et al. (1992) and Dijkers (1997) report similar research findings for persons with spinal cord injuries.

Quality of life judgments are highly individualized; they vary over time and even from day to day.

Just as dialysis machines represent a lifeline for people with end stage renal disease, individuals with severe cerebral palsy or with a spinal cord injury have found assistive technologies and personal assistance to be important lifelines for achieving a higher quality of life. Continued study of people's satisfaction with personal assistance shows a strong relationship with overall life satisfaction (Nosek, Fuhrer, & Potter, 1995), yet as these researchers note, the nature of that desired lifeline is individualized:

Personal assistance is a complex issue for persons with disabilities, varying from person to person in the amount of assistance needed, preferences for how a task is done, and attitudes toward a disability and the resulting need for assistance (p. 201).

Assistive devices, too, present individuals with complex choices around which they can exercise individual preferences. Thus, satisfaction with both AT and personal assistance is individualized and difficult to measure. Quality of life, satisfaction with personal assistance, and satisfaction with assistive devices are dynamic constructs. Not only can each change over time, thereby redefining the other constructs, but their collective relationship is dynamic because individuals age, develop new strengths and skills, and so on. This relationship is complex and often difficult for either the individual with a disability or the professional to assess.

Ann and Linda, 1986

In 1981, two women with severe cerebral palsy were feeling they had a poor quality of life. Ann, age 42, was ambulatory but with unintelligible speech; Linda, age 52, used a wheelchair and had more intelligible, yet slow, speech. They were both residents of a nursing home where the conditions were "deteriorating badly." It was becoming physically run down and the quality of the care was poor. According to them,

> The attendants couldn't speak English and our speech is not good so there was no communication. Also, we had no privacy. Men, women, anyone would just walk in at any time. They treated us like non-persons and I guess they felt that you can't intrude on a non-person. We were going crazy just trying to stay sane.

Linda had been in that nursing home for thirteen years and Ann for ten. Finally, out of desperation, they thought that together they might be able to live in an apartment, providing they could get daily personal assistance. But that proved to be quite a challenge:

> We couldn't get out of the Home until we got an aide, and we couldn't get an aide because we were in a nursing home.

Eventually, they found personal assistance for four hours, six days a week to bathe and shower them and to cook and clean their apartment. Taking it one day at a time, they tried new things and gradually became more and more independent. Ann says, "Since I've been here I've been able to do a lot more on my own."

Ann found that more frequent interactions and communication helped improve her speech; Linda agrees and adds that their ongoing communication helped "sharpen her hearing" so that she understood more of what Ann was saying. Gradually, Ann stopped using her communication board.

Now I just use it when people don't understand me. Places like the doctor's office where it's important for people to understand me. It's really a last resort. I know myself and when I get anxious I can't talk. I still use it sometimes with Linda to spell out an uncommon word, but it's very slow and Linda's eyes get tired. We've both learned how to relax — my mouth and Linda's ears both have calmed down.

Ann was always more ambulatory than Linda, but found herself using a manual wheelchair more and more. Linda, however, wanted and needed the enhanced control offered by a power chair. This technology presented her with both opportunities for mobility and problems:

I was trying for over three years to get a new wheelchair. It broke down all the time. One day I was going to the store with my attendant and it just stopped in the middle of the sidewalk. They had to go back and borrow Ann's chair for me to use. Three days later I got a loaner. I had to have that accident before I got the new chair. If it wasn't for that, I'd probably still have that old chair.

Ann and Linda had a tendency to be cautious about venturing out by themselves, but that incident with Linda's power chair heightened their concern about getting stranded. When I asked them about using the special vans for wheelchairs provided by their city's public transit authority, they said,

It's difficult to go out. Transportation is a big problem. They pick you up but to get back home again is unpredictable. We are afraid of going out and getting stranded. Especially in bad weather.

Both Ann and Linda had resolved, however, to conquer their hesitations and limitations and become even more independent. To them, there were many opportunities just waiting to be discovered. As Linda said,

Like everyone, we strive for more, for the highest we can get. What is life without striving for more?

When I talked with them in 1988, they had experienced the typical ups and downs in transportation, personal assistance, and assistive technology use, but they seemed to feel more in control of their lives. They had taken a trip to Disney World and Epcot Center and found they could leave their apartment — and even their city — and enjoy traveling and exploring new areas. Nine years after leaving the nursing home, they had achieved a quality of life personally satisfying to themselves, as their 1990 Christmas letter indicates:

Merry Christmas and Happy New Year to all relatives and friends. Hope this has been a good year for all of you. And the coming year will be even better.

This has been a pretty good year for us considering everything. The Good Lord continues to bless us with the strength to go on. And for this we are very grateful. We are going on our ninth year in our apartment. Needless to say we are very proud of ourselves.

We did lose our adopted mother and angel Mary, who took care of us for over four years. However once again The Good Lord was with us, as He proved He has more than one angel. We now have Mary's daughter Tracey, who is just wonderful.

This was the first summer since we've been in our apartment that we did not go any place. But you might say we had a vacation right at home. Since we both have electric wheelchairs now, it makes it a lot easier to get around. Up until this summer we were both afraid to cross the street alone. However, one Sunday morning Linda said to me, "Let's cross the street." So I followed. We found out it was not as hard as we thought. After that there was no keeping us home. A lot of our days were spent riding around our beautiful neighborhood. We felt like two birds who could get up and fly whenever we felt like it.

One of the highlights of our summer was a visit from three of Linda's nephews who live in New Mexico. John and Raymond spent a week with us in August. It was so nice to be able to offer them a place to stay. Having them here was like a vacation for us, too. We all spent one day at the Museum of Science and Industry. This was really a treat after not being there for so many years. We walked to the Zoo twice, which is about four blocks from where we live. John found the most accessible way to go with the wheelchairs. So we took about three trips by ourselves after that. Linda even made it alone one day. During our week with John and Raymond we also had a ninetieth birthday party for Uncle Fred, who has since then passed away. What a beautiful way to remember him.

During the later part of October, Dave surprised us by coming in for a convention. He was able to spend one Sunday evening with us. And came back the next morning for breakfast.

We've had a few visits from our good friend Lois. Even though she moved back to Indiana, she makes [our city] her second home, and does visit us each time she comes in.

Bob continues to be an adopted brother, and is so helpful — taking us to plays, shows, and a lot of places we never dreamed we'd get.

Richard has become a real brother. Quite often he will spend the weekend with us. He will do a lot of things for us. We will either order out, or go out and eat. Then have a lot of fun playing five hundred rummy.

This will tell you a little bit about what's going on with the Rainbow connection. All good wishes for Christmas and the coming year.

Ann

Linda

Ann and Linda's letter indicates that they are leading full and satisfying lives. Yet their experiences highlight several problems some people with disabilities have today living independently.

Knowledge of and comfort with technology. As women, and in particular women born with disabilities, they were not brought up to feel knowledgeable about machines and technical devices and, thus, did not feel completely comfortable with them. It is evident that only recently have they been able to trust that their wheelchairs will not leave them stranded. Their initial cautiousness kept them from pursuing some opportunities earlier, and others they have yet to pursue. In spite of the opportunities assistive technologies afford them, even making their independence possible, their devices initially presented new challenges. Coming as these challenges did in the midst of other changes in their lives, they no doubt seemed all the more daunting. Yet they received little or no training in or preparation for their use, and it was gradually, through trial and error, that they learned to use them to their benefit.

Lack of incentives for older persons' enhanced independence. Ann and Linda were never given the chance to be either "normal" children or "normal" adults. Now chronologically middle aged, but almost childlike in their eagerness for friendship and to learn and experience what has been until recently unavailable to them, they appear at times to be caught between mature and youthful identities. Older persons with developmental disabilities have special needs that are starting only now to be recognized.

In spite of their consistent efforts to develop and increase their capabilities, their ages make them unattractive to many vocational rehabilitation programs and, thus, the traditional societal rewards for an enhanced level of functioning (job training, education, employment) are not available to them. It is their strong desire to live outside of a nursing home that serves as their primary motivation for their independence. Additional motivation comes from their desire for new experiences and a full life.

Difficulties in obtaining personal assistance. Devoid of money, consistent family help, and job skills, not having had experience with such basics as finding a job and a place to live, the odds were against Ann's and Linda's success in living on their own. Through their ingenuity and persistence, however, and with the help of friends and a number of shared personal assistants, they are succeeding. The primary payback for their continued independence — and a very significant one to them — is not having to return to a nursing home. Yet continuous frustrations in obtaining reliable personal assistance are frequent reminders that many of their gains could be lost if the desired level of help and support is not available.

Maggie, 1991

Until recently, people with severe chronic illnesses or physical disabilities typically did not live far into older adulthood. Now many elderly parents anguish over who will take care of their children after their deaths. And their children are very concerned themselves, as Jim mentioned when talking about his friend Nancy:

> She thinks about her mother dying, and she wants to die with her mother because nobody will take care of her.

Maggie, first discussed in Chapter Two, has had a considerable functional decline. She and her caretaker, Theresa, moved back to Maggie's hometown to be close to family and friends. Maggie's example illustrates some additional problems aging persons with disabilities often must confront.

I had not heard from Maggie in over a year until one Sunday night I received a phone call from Theresa. Since Maggie had lost her job with the Independent Living Center in early 1987 ("I didn't learn my responsibilities fast enough — I grew up in a world that didn't teach me how to handle responsibilities — plus I had personality conflicts with my boss"), she had been doing volunteer work helping special education students in a public school. Now, Theresa informed me, Maggie had been in and out of hospitals and rehabilitation facilities for most of the past year. Maggie had surgery on her neck that left her paralyzed from the neck down. As Maggie herself later wrote,

> It started off with loss of function in my left arm and hand, the two most important appendages of my body as I used them for pointing, directing my motorized wheelchair, holding Theresa while she transferred me, and many more things which I took for granted. It ended about eight months later with the loss of function of my legs.

Because of Maggie's changed condition, she and Theresa moved back to Maggie's hometown "to be close to family and friends." Maggie's mother, who had been living in the same apartment complex until "she kept falling" because of back problems, moved with them. Concern over the welfare of Maggie's mother added to the share of the burden Theresa feels she carries. As Maggie herself puts it,

Theresa is doing extremely well considering all she has been through with me, especially the move that she was not too happy about. She had spent almost every night with me in the hospitals and had spent every night at Memorial with me, so she just wanted things to be normal again. I, on the other hand, became extremely depressed because the only activity I could engage in was to think of all of what I used to do. There are times now, though, when I think she has accepted my new disability better than I have — or did until the past few months. Before I got my new wheelchair she would say, "Things will get better when your wheelchair comes" and "We will just have to struggle through it like I said before your surgery."

Maggie now needs new assistive technologies because her condition has changed so much. Both Maggie and Theresa needed to get used to these changes, which added more stress to what each was already feeling.

After my neurologist ordered an MRI, it turns out I have what is called a swan neck deformity. When I put my head forward my spine closes and the fluid stops flowing. When I put it up, the fluid starts again. I came home with a cervical collar and a corset — more for support than for correcting the problem, as the doctors assured me I couldn't get any worse.

Everyone was holding their breath when my motorized, reclining wheelchair arrived as I could still sit up when the seat and back were made and the chair was ordered. To everyone's relief, the doctor said I didn't need either the cervical collar or my corset when I used the wheelchair. I was especially glad, as I didn't like to look that disabled, or you could say, I wasn't accustomed to having that many people stare at me. Even though I've had a disability life, little did I know that the new chair would really cause people to stare — but more out of amazement than pity. The chair itself is the optimum in high-tech. It is all controlled by using a joystick that I hold in my mouth. This enables me to be in the recliner mode, the drive mode, and the Light Talker mode, meaning I can use my communication device in this mode. I change modes by pushing a button at the side of my head. People have said it looks like a rocket, especially when I'm tilted all the way back.

Luckily, there was a one-time grant given through the state and people from UCPA [the United Cerebral Palsy Association] suggested I apply. It and Medicaid paid for the wheelchair. It paid less than one-fourth of the cost of the Light Talker [a sophisticated communication device which evolved from earlier products such as her Express III]. Fortunately, I bought the van before all this happened, or there would have been the additional expense of purchasing one and having it customized. Without it, I would be stuck at home as it is impossible to get my chair in a car. Mother helped pay for the Light Talker that gives me a means of communication.

UCPA has a program to teach people how to use an IBM computer and then find employment for them. I am going to enter it in early '92 as, if I can, I would like to have a part-time job writing or doing something along those lines. Anyway, it will do me good to learn more about IBMs and to know that I may be able to become productive again.

Maggie's experience illustrates some additional challenges in helping aging persons with physical disabilities maintain their quality of life:

Added stress on already burdened caretakers. Family members and other caretakers who devote a major portion of their day to the care of the person with a disability may feel overwhelmed by the heightened need for medical and technological interventions. When, in spite of such assistance, they see the individual continue to deteriorate or become depressed, they may experience their own sense of helplessness and despair.

New device and equipment needs. Aging persons with disabilities undergo changes in their physical capabilities and general health that require modifications in devices and heightened attention to their special needs. Maggie illustrates this, and so does Chuck. In 1991, Chuck had been in intensive care after a severe case of bronchitis. "My carbon dioxide level was high and now I need to be on oxygen all the time." Yet he tries to get out as much as possible, and says: "When I'm out shopping or go out to eat I don't use the oxygen."

Rehabilitation professionals and the designers of assistive technologies will increasingly need to address functional declines in aging persons with disabilities, and the preservation of as much previous functioning as possible.

To summarize, there is a complex interactive relationship among assistive device use, quality of life, functional capabilities, and temperament, and this relationship can change over time. Therefore, this entire constellation of factors needs to be continually addressed, first from a person-centered perspective, and secondarily from a functional, disability-centered one.

Key to appreciating how — and why — some people with disabilities attain a highly satisfying quality of life, while others do not, is understanding the various ways individuals strive to satisfy personal needs and establish an identity in today's society. It is to these topics that I turn in Chapter Eight.

Footnotes Chapter Six

[1] Quality of life: In *Outcomes Following Traumatic Spinal Cord Injury: Clinical Practice Guidelines for Health-Care Professionals* (Consortium for Spinal Cord Medicine, 1999), quality of life is defined as: "a personal, global, evaluation of well-being or general satisfaction with life experienced by people under their current life conditions" (p. 24).

CHAPTER SEVEN

Myths and Machines

> *There is some Myth for every man, which if we but knew it,*
> *would make us understand all he did and thought.*
> — **WILLIAM BUTLER YEATS**

We are often so taken with the potential benefits of assistive devices for persons with disabilities that we fail to fully consider the quality of life of the individuals who will use these technologies. *Quality of life* considerations require focused attention on a person's *desired* achievement psychologically, socially, intellectually, and vocationally in spite of limitations in physical functioning. All too often, however, the emphasis is on the physical aspects to the near exclusion of other needs, such as the user's social and emotional needs. This chapter discusses the ways in which people come to terms with life with a physical disability. Often individuals respond in ways that are derived from learned patterns for need satisfaction, their personality characteristics, and the expectations others have of them. These responses produce hope in some individuals and despair in others. This inclination toward either hope or despair influences a person's view of opportunities, growth, and the use of technological and other assistance, and ultimately determines his or her *disability experience* and quality of life.

Carolyn Vash (1981), a psychologist with tetraplegia, indicates that three main factors are related to defining a person's *disability experience* and each is relevant to the current discussion:

1. *Physiological Factors (Physical Condition of the Self): The Nature of the Disability as Determining the Disability Experience*. Varying states of health can lead to different complications and sequelae, courses of treatment, and rehabilitation. They also determine a person's energy level and physical comfort (pain, heat tolerance, etc.). Functioning also depends on the extent to which the environment permits the highest quality care (e.g., placement in a rehabilitation center equipped with the most advanced interventions and ATs).

2. *Psychosocial Factors (The Attitudes and Responses of Others): Environmental and Social Determinants of the Disability Experience*. The attitudes and responses of others, expressed by the interactions within the family or through exposure to the responses

of others (employers, coworkers, teachers, and so on) can have a profound influence on the person with a disability. Self-concept, motivation, and personal aspirations of an individual may be shaped by social interactions that influence perspectives of resources and opportunities.

A person's social support network (family, friends, personal assistants, work colleagues, etc.) can greatly affect the *disability experience* and may even influence daily functioning and rehabilitation outcomes. Social support systems strongly influence how people with disabilities interpret their experiences and evaluate their options. To illustrate: There is a strong deaf culture at the National Technical Institute for the Deaf in Rochester, New York. The student peer group has a great influence on individual student decisions regarding whether or not to use technologies for sound amplification. This network may not only affect what alternatives the person with a disability views as available, but can affect one's sense of well-being and even health status. It is also the case that the ways in which rehabilitation professionals define the disability experience and rehabilitation success are potent environmental influences on individuals with disabilities.

3. *Psychological Factors (Attitudes Of and Toward the Self): Individual Differences as Determinants of the Disability Experience.* As we have seen, people with disabilities — even the same disability — have different ideas about their own limitations and capabilities. They vary in their views of what living with a disability is like and in their course of adjustment to the disability. Their temperaments and ways of coping with the persons and situations in their lifespace are factors influencing such differences.

In addition to typologies such as Vash's, other psychological theories can help to develop an understanding of the roots of depression, anxiety, anger, substance abuse, loneliness, social isolation, and other phenomena experienced by a number of persons who have cerebral palsy or a spinal cord injury. A discussion follows regarding how different people are motivated to satisfy their needs and to use assistive technologies — or not.

Motivation to Meet Needs

Abraham Maslow (1954) theorized that human beings develop according to a hierarchy of five levels of needs, graphically depicted in a pyramidal form as in Figure 7-1. He ranked these needs in the order

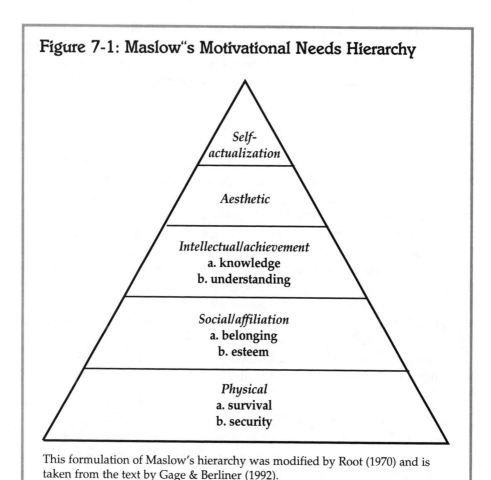

Figure 7-1: Maslow"s Motivational Needs Hierarchy

Self-
actualization

Aesthetic

Intellectual/achievement
a. knowledge
b. understanding

Social/affiliation
a. belonging
b. esteem

Physical
a. survival
b. security

This formulation of Maslow's hierarchy was modified by Root (1970) and is taken from the text by Gage & Berliner (1992).

in which individuals satisfied them, beginning with the most basic at the bottom of the pyramid and working upward. Maslow maintained that needs must be met at each successive level before one moves on to higher levels — beginning with the most basic, *physical needs*, then to *social needs*, and so on. The drive to satisfy these needs is *motivation*. That is, what motivates us to perform particular behaviors, persevere, complete tasks, and take risks is the need to feel secure, to belong, to achieve, etc. Maslow's motivational needs hierarchy suggests that there must be a "psychological readiness" (or satisfaction of lower level needs) before one can be expected to be motivated to move up the hierarchy. Frustrated needs result in anger and/or anxiety, which, if turned inward, may lead to depression.

Maslow's theory illustrates common attributes of a developmental theory. Persons successfully develop and adjust to ever more complex behaviors as they live and grow in a widening range of areas and build on successful earlier achievements. It is easy to see this growth when one compares and contrasts the complexity of behaviors evident among adults with those among children. When a young adult who once functioned at the higher levels receives a traumatic injury (such as a spinal cord injury), he or she has to re-focus again on the satisfaction of more basic physical needs. Such adults often find themselves having to go through each successive stage again, meeting their needs for affiliation with new friends and achievement needs in an entirely different career area than originally planned.

In a parallel fashion, when a person grows up with cerebral palsy and his or her life situation is sharply altered by assistive devices so that once-impossible tasks can be performed independently, that person is changed. The person's desires and drives also may change. This is the focus of the next sections; they examine situations from the perspective of Jim, a person who has attained a high level of functioning, but wants and yearns for more — plainly, he wants it all!

Individuals need to feel connected to the world in which they live — connected to other people, connected to a social role — to feel that they matter and that their lives are meaningful.

BEYOND BASIC NEEDS

Jim, 1988, Continued

Jim was becoming a "reluctant user" of assistive devices and had a growing desire to do things without them. In 1988, he said, "I've been walking around a lot lately and I'm getting run down and worn out physically."

The physical toll on him is one thing, the emotional another. The man I talked with in 1988 had become quite different from the one I had met two years before.

> I met a woman who works in a bar I was hanging out in. Since I walked in, she only saw me sitting there at the table like anyone else. She didn't know I use a wheelchair. So without knowing that, she invited me out for a drink. But then when she saw me get in my wheelchair, she made some excuse for not being able to go out, for being tired. It just blew her mind.

Jim had related several anecdotes that had involved him in bars. I was becoming concerned that Jim might be developing a dependence on alcohol. I didn't want to sound confrontational, so I adopted a more indirect approach. "Even though you can do everything at work that your colleagues do, it still sometimes takes twice or three times as long, so that frustration and physical exhaustion can set in. A lot of people in that situation either drink too much or use drugs. I was wondering if you would know why and what can be done about that?"

> I think I drink too much. It helps me to unwind and maybe to deal with my frustrations. It's probably a little bit of both. I drink a lot more during the week but I think the only regret I have, in order for me to relax, is companionship. I feel I'm normal in every way but in companionship. I think it's the emptiness.
> It's not the lack of opportunity, it's the lack of confidence. In my family, we just don't talk that much. I never learned how to express myself and to be less passive.
> My friend says I live in a dream world, and he is making me aware of how I try to make a fairy tale life out of a relationship and I've got to stop doing that so I don't get hurt.

Jim now finds himself caught in several dilemmas: Thanks to the rehabilitation services he received, he was trained for a job that he likes and has succeeded in. His co-workers treat him as both a colleague and friend and try to help and further socialize him. He is trying very hard to form an identity as a "normal person," and he finds it difficult to tolerate the company of other people with disabilities similar to his own.

Yet Jim's vocational success has led to his desire for equality on other dimensions for which his prior socialization did not prepare him. Jim's continual striving, developing identity, and physical exhaustion have taken an emotional toll on him to the point where he seems to be frustrated, insecure, and depressed — which he largely attributes to the attitudes and faults of others.

Jim's confused identity also led him to make some rather poor judgments. By not using his assistive devices regularly, he became physically run-down. He interpreted the motives and actions of others in a defensive manner; for example, he perceived his difficulties in relating to other people with disabilities as being due to their shortcomings:" I get interesting vibes from other handicapped people. They are embarrassed for my success because it makes them look lazy." As seen in Chapter Six, when his father inquired into his financial health, it was not because of Jim's inability to handle money, but because of his father's overprotectiveness and lack of confidence in Jim's capabilities.

The following statement shows that Jim also ascribes to his father feelings which the father has projected onto his other children.

> My dad wants to repay my brothers and sisters for the shame they endured because of me, when we were younger and they were ashamed to have their friends over. But they themselves say they've never felt ashamed.

When asked about Jim's "identity crisis," his speech therapist provided the following:

> Compared to persons in sheltered work situations, Jim gets along beautifully. But when he's out in the community, people are not comparing him to people in sheltered workshops, they're comparing him to his non-disabled colleagues.
>
> Often, by increasing individuals' functioning to an almost non-disabled level, it may occur that these same individuals can't deal with the frustrations they've suddenly been faced with. Many people have very unrealistic expectations. We see it in parents, employers, vocational rehabilitation counselors, speech therapists, the physicians here. Many people think that once that person has the appropriate technology, that the problem is going to be solved and that the person is going to be "normal." It's just not true.

Another rehabilitation professional concurs:

> Someone who is very high functioning cognitively is very aware of what the rest of the world out there is like. They have an 'I am really different' perspective. They may look at others and say, "Boy, wouldn't it be great to be that way." They may have had a fantasy of wishing to be like everyone else. When they see a good deal of progress towards normalcy, they tend to overexpect things to happen as a result. Employers, everyone, now are expecting more as well. But often it's a whole new world of frustrations that opens. Mobility may no longer be a frustration, but relationships are.
>
> We all cope with frustrations in our lives according to how we've coped in the past. People with CP have had much more limited experiences to garner [good] coping strategies and, with such dramatic changes now available to them — probably more than the average person will ever experience — plus real physical limitations, the emotional experiences and anxieties can be tough.

The optimism around the elimination of functional limitations has led to higher expectations on the part of some families, professionals and employers. Perhaps no higher expectations exist than those individuals with disabilities often have for themselves. Jim's example continues to be illustrative:

Jim, 1991

The first thing Jim said to me when I called to tell him I was going to be in his city for a conference was, "Guess what? My picture is being shown all over the world."

We had agreed to meet one late afternoon in the lobby of the conference center. Then he suggested we go to a bar, saying, "In this city after work, you can get a free dinner from the snacks served in the bars."

Jim was dressed in a navy blue striped shirt, red tie, and light blue suit. He had loosened his tie, like other men in the bar who had just left work.

As soon as we were seated, he showed me the cover of his company's annual report. There he was, front and center, and around him were a couple of older workers and members of a variety of cultures. Again, he talked about his international exposure.

Then Jim brought me up to date on his family. His father died in January 1990 of cancer — he had been sick for close to two years. In that time, Jim drove to visit him almost every weekend. At the same time, he was in a car pool and would take other people to work. "All told, I put about 50,000 miles on my van in one year."

Jim had to sell his condo because he fell two months behind on his payments, which he attributed to traveling so often to be with his father. They told him he either had to pay the entire remaining balance or give up the condo. He had to do the latter and now lives in an apartment downtown.

Jim is so financially strapped that he is also in the process of selling his van. Now that he lives downtown, he can get to work on his scooter and says he only needs to drive his van about once a week. When he gets the money from the sale of his van, he wants to go to Las Vegas.

Then he talked about how things were going at work. He was disappointed with his most recent raise, and said that people have told him that he's not paid well. I asked about the prospects for a promotion, and he said, "Not in the near future. If someone offered me a better paying job, I'd take it." I had the impression that he felt his company should pay him more in exchange for the privilege of being able to feature an employee in a powered scooter on the cover of their annual report. I then asked him about returning to school to finish his degree. Jim answered, "It's hard after working all day with computers and ledger sheets and books to do more with that."

He said he leads an active social life and added that his interest in being around people with disabilities is just about completely gone now. Then Jim told me, "Ten weeks and one day ago my heart was broken" by a woman who was a cocktail waitress and model. They had been going out for about six months. He talked about the movies they had seen and that he had taken her out for dinner on numerous occasions. Then she suddenly told him that she no longer wanted to see him.

The last couple of months, he says, have been very rough on him. He wants a romantic relationship but feels very discouraged about having one soon. He said that people with disabilities are not seen as desirable sexual partners and gave an example of going to a "striptease place, one I often visit, where the dancers do a routine with the men but they wouldn't with me."

We had been talking for over an hour when Jim suddenly announced that he had forgotten something at work that he needed to have that evening. He finished his drink and, without having any of the snacks they served, paid the bill. As we were making our way back out, he told me that he is very glad he was able to be with his father when he died, and to be with him through his long illness. But he's sad that his father died without knowing how capable he is. And his mother is still in the process of becoming aware of his capabilities. Then he said that one of his sisters has a habit of "popping in" on him and cleaning his apartment and bringing him groceries. While he loves his sister, he clearly interpreted her caretaking as "patronizing" and said once again that "My family just doesn't trust my capabilities."

Relationship Rehabilitation: "Mobility may no longer be a frustration, but relationships are"

Maslow's need for affiliation is compatible with Norris Hansell's (1974) analysis of our essential attachments to the world in which we live — a connection to other persons, a social role, to the feeling one matters and that one's life is meaningful and has vitality. In keeping with Maslow, let us consider another hierarchy. One we will call a *relationship hierarchy*. In a sense, it is a fine-grained analysis of social/affiliation needs.

The richness and variety of relationships we have is what comes to define us over time as individuals. When we are infants, our first and strongest relationships are typically with our parents. To thrive, we need to jump in at the top two layers or blocks and trust and love them. When we are mature, we begin at the first relationship building block to form new alliances and friendships. Traditionally, our initial attraction to someone else (physical appearance, personality, and so on) continues when we discover we are compatible and have shared values and interests (recreational, cultural, vocational, sexual, financial, generational).

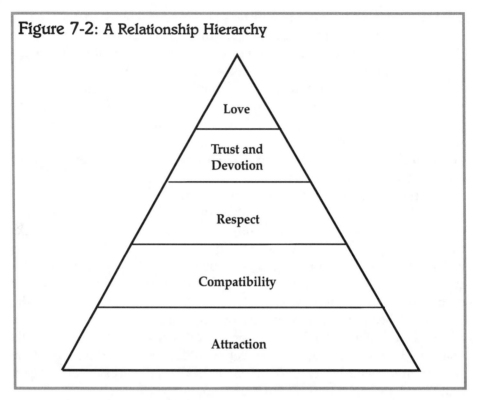

Figure 7-2: A Relationship Hierarchy

Love

Trust and Devotion

Respect

Compatibility

Attraction

A lot can be learned about the steps in which relationships form by watching college students. Over the course of a year, in the living laboratory of a college campus, we observe freshman in their attempts to form alliances, to fit in and belong, by adopting a particular dress code and selecting a particular group to join. The peer group affiliation, even more than academic success, leads to a sense of a good match with a particular college environment. In fact, this is the most crucial factor in college retention (e.g., Stinson, Scherer & Walter, 1988).

The respect for one another as unique individuals with separate needs and preferences, and the formation of trust and devotion, is what leads to loving another person. This is what marriages are built upon. Over time, there may be imbalances in compatibility as educational or career paths shift and life stresses occur with each partner dealing with those stresses in different ways. There can also be lapses in trust and devotion. Brian discussed many of these points when he updated me on his relationship with a woman from Japan:

> We're no longer together, but we were for over a year and it was probably one of the best relationships I've had. She knew what my needs were and she met those. She had needs, too, and I accommodated those. We lived

together about 9 months, but it was challenging… there's definitely pros and cons to every relationship. … at least when she was living here she didn't have to pay rent and she was able to save up for nursing school.

She is from Japan and on a student visa for 5 years She was in a nursing student program and to do it financially she needed to get married, and wanted to get married, and I just couldn't do that. A lot depended on finances, and her need to do things and be independent. Also, she was pretty young, 26 years old. But we were really good for each other.

She was determined and very strong but she had a lot of weak points, too. My love for her was to a point where I don't want to cage in a bird that needs to fly and it was for me a need for more independence and not being so needy. She is very traditional Japanese. She didn't like me having women friends. We spent a little bit too much time together.

All relationships undergo stress. How the difficulties and strain are acknowledged and dealt with will determine whether or not a relationship continues. A marriage continues when a rebalance of the relationship elements is achieved. But if one or more of the above building blocks completely disintegrates, the marriage will likely come apart.

Our relationships so define us that the number and quality of relationships a person has becomes an important diagnostic criterion for personality disorders and psychopathology. Children who are devoid of trusting and loving relationships often having difficulties forming appropriate bonds with others in adulthood. Individuals who have been emotionally and physically abused — regardless of age — similarly have difficulties, especially with trust.

A major part of developing and maturing is learning the proper formation, maintenance and nurturing of relationships, which can remain elusive for many people. Like Jim, many individuals born with a disability haven't had the depth and breadth of social encounters to learn sophisticated relationship skills. This can have lifelong consequences as was stated to me by a colleague who feels very strongly about the need for attention to social skills. She is both a social worker and a rehabilitation counselor in Chicago, and is blind:

> The learned behavior is negatively influenced by well-intentioned family, friends, and professionals who allow inappropriate social actions due to the person's disability. This unfortunate allowance only serves to perpetuate poor social skills. In turn this well-intentioned allowance further widens the possibility of unsuccessful relationships later.
>
> Professionals as well as family members must become educated to having expectations that are appropriate for people with disabilities. It is not at all helpful to make allowances in behavior unless the disability is cognitive in nature. It should be a part of the rehabilitation process that

any consumer who utilizes systemic help be assessed for appropriate social skills functioning. I know that Centers for Independent Living exist, however a great many of the disabled staff are used to the inappropriate social interaction, especially if they have spent much of their life surrounded by other people with disabilities. I am appalled by the lack of intervention in this area. It is in my estimation even more important then work rehabilitation, because the most skilled employee is not going to work in a vacuum.

If a disability was acquired in early adulthood, old relationships may fade and new ones need to be found, as both Brian and Butch experienced. The lack of desired and quality relationships can lead to depression, further social withdrawal and decreased social participation. Regardless if the person was born with a disability or acquired one, many times the individual thinks the lack of appropriate relationships are due to the disability and physical attraction when that may not be the case. Compatibility factors (shared interests and values, having a likeable and sociable personality, etc,) are more often than not what makes the difference. This was discussed by Brian when he and I had a conversation about his current relationships:

> **B:** Right now, lots of people who were in my life have moved on to other states, to pursue careers, get married.
> **M:** You've lost a big part of your circle.
>
> **B:** I've had to re-establish old relationships and form new ones. My best friend has moved and has a girlfriend and he hasn't called me in 3-4 months. Relationships are very important. But so is having time to yourself. You need to find a good balance. I find it easier to be by myself than to explain myself to other people.
>
> **M:** In 1986, a major goal for you was to get married.
>
> **B:** I was living at home and thought it would be great to have someone like my mom take care of me everyday like this. But someone my own age or younger doing this. Getting out on my own, I've found it's a lot more difficult than that. I don't know if I'm much of a relationships kind of person. I've had quite a few over the years and they're a lot of work. I see different partnerships in disabled relationships and it's tough to stay together.
>
> **M:** What makes it tough?
>
> **B:** It's doing the things the other person wants to do. The combinations are endless as far as the feelings and interests in each partner. Going out

versus staying at home, which restaurant to go to, and all that. There's one couple, he's a quad, and he's very needy. They're lifelong partners and married a long time. They just recently broke up. She was trapped in his world. He treated her like a slave. They needed and should have arranged for care providers.

M: You make sure your relationships are more shared, give-and take.

B: Why is it so hard for me to juggle a girlfriend, or establish a relationship? Why is that such a stumbling block? Is it because I'm old? Because I'm in a wheelchair? Is it because I'm not exciting enough? What is it that's blocking my view of wanting to establish another relationship? These are all intriguing. I've been dealt a set of circumstances that … I know I won't get married in this lifetime and the ones who are most special to me now are my care providers. The ones who come over and help me with my daily needs and wipe my butt. They're special people and a lot of them are woman. I have male providers, too, but the women are the motherly type that can deal with that kind of stuff. So they're there for me and we're able to share our lives in the morning and at night. One of my care providers, she's a mom and a very kind-hearted person, said to me, "You're going to have so many more people come into your life. You're still young and you'll have just as many more people come into your life as you've had already." What's interesting is, wow, who are these people going to be? I'll be meeting new people who will give me new ideas, give me new insights, and take me in new directions.

As has been discussed throughout this book, people with disabilities want to participate in society as much as and equally with everyone else. It may not be so much the barriers related to the disability and the environment that stand in their way (although they certainly can be significant obstacles), but the barriers to relationships that exist. It may not be so much a physical or a disability issue as a compatibility one. As we have moved from a medical model to a social model of rehabilitation, and as we now value social participation as the key outcome of rehabilitation services, this is where we need to put much more focused attention.

How does one make the choice about when to use AT and when to seek assistance from another person? While AT helps to break down physical barriers to social participation and relationships, some ATs can be barriers to interpersonal contact. An emphasis needs to be placed on interpersonal communication skills and relationship formation and maintenance. Like Jim, some people with disabilities struggle with, for example:

- balancing independence, interdependence, and often unavoidable dependence

- knowing what to share, just how much, when and with whom

- learning ways to convey needs and preferences in a manner that preserves self-esteem and respects the needs, preferences, and feelings of others

- managing social interactions in the context of pain, fatigue, the need to do things in different ways and at particular times

- anticipating what may occur in social encounters as well as preparing strategies for handling the unexpected

- tempering reactions and knowing when to use humor, when to be serious and frank and when to just listen and not respond

Building interpersonal relationship skills can seem a complex and even formidable task, especially when one lacks self-confidence and esteem. Each of the individuals in this book have made statements indicating that they struggle with the management of relationships. For many people with disabilities, *relationship rehabilitation* is needed. This is an area where thousands of peer role models exist and should be sought out and encouraged to work with less experienced persons with disabilities. They can be found in workplaces throughout the world, on the boards of directors of many organizations, in politics, education, and medicine — in short, everywhere. Unlike the "super crips" that have often become a target of resentment, these individuals are quietly going about leading successful lives. Supportive peer groups in independent living centers could also make an important impact by fostering open discussions of relationship issues, building confidence, and providing opportunities to try out, practice and role play new skills. Finally, there are many publications and web sites (see Appendix C) where relationship questions are frequently addressed.

Beyond Companionship to Sexual Expression

For Jim, having a job has turned out to be an incomplete victory. He now is striving to attain the skills and confidence to cope with all of life's opportunities and challenges, and the chance to fall in love — to develop an intimate relationship. He had said in 1986,

> Recently, though, I've started to think... I've been too busy with my independence to go out and relax, to date. So now I'm alone. I feel it is time to have [an intimate] relationship. I realized I wasn't going to do it where I work because if you go the handicapped route you're not exposed to too

many handicapped people there, and when you are, it doesn't work out the way it's supposed to. But with AB's [able-bodied persons] I can't go so fast. [With one girl in particular:] It's hard for me to get out my feelings... I've been too busy with my handicap to know what that's all about....

[Later he added:] I'm struggling and striving for what? To live alone? There's a beautiful girl out there... Every time I give up something positive happens. Like when I gave up on trying to drive. And I gave up on a job.

Jim's confusion about wanting a relationship with another "handicapped" person or with an "able-bodied" woman is not unusual. A similar dilemma was heard from Ken, who at the time had a live-in girlfriend:

As far as living with somebody or getting married, I could never marry, I don't think, another disabled person or somebody in a wheelchair. Friendship-wise, it's split about half-half. But as far as a relationship, I just can't picture being with somebody I depend so much on. It would just be too many hassles. It'd be cumbersome physically, and emotionally also. I think a lot of times, too, there's a trade-off. She helps out more in the physical part, I help out more on the emotional part. [With another person with a disability] there'd be no trading-off, it wouldn't be complementary. But as far as identifying, sometimes both, sometimes in-between and sometimes neither.

Most of the individuals with physical disabilities in this study said they were very lonely; that they desired physical contact and intimacy, to have their bodies be accepted in a romantic or sexual way. For example, Chuck talked about wanting to meet women but believed that they have "a tendency to move away from me... It's hard to approach somebody when you're in a wheelchair, as opposed to the way it was before." Brian, too, when expressing his wish for a girlfriend, said: "It would be all that much... more." Maggie wishes she had "more of a social life."

In an article titled "Not a Fifth Wheel: Sexual Expression Needs to be Mainstreamed, Too," William Rush (1985), a 28 year-old journalist with cerebral palsy, believes that his "struggle for self-sufficiency has been so significant that a relationship at this time is out of the question." Echoing the sentiments of Jim, Ken, Chuck, and Brian, he goes on to say how hard it is to get to know people, especially if you're shy, and that power wheelchairs prevent people with disabilities from getting close to anyone.

And when I'm bent over my letterboard or voice synthesizer, spelling thoughts out with my headstick, I can't establish eye contact.

His cerebral palsy is the type that results in uncontrollable muscle spasms:

> I can't put my arms around a woman without the risk of giving her a black eye.

While he realizes his body "is far from perfect," he notes that when it comes to sexual expression, society does not perceive adults with cerebral palsy as interested participants or as desirable partners, viewing them more as "eternal children" than as sexual beings and potential love partners. People with cerebral palsy have masculine and feminine identities which influence their relations in general, and Rush states, in line with Maslow's theory, that intimate relationships are needed "because we would be incomplete and unable to live totally alone. We need companionship and to care about others and to be cared for and about." With a determined, somewhat angry tone, he adds,

> My problem is not faulty equipment... I know I'm capable of loving and being loved. And I'm tired of being told I can be independent while being denied the chance of being interdependent; I'm tired of being told I have so much to offer society while being denied the opportunity of giving my love to another person.

Like Jim, many persons with disabilities have succeeded in becoming employed in competitive jobs. Their need for accomplishment is well served, but affiliation needs are not given nearly as much attention in their education and training. According to Maslow and Erikson, this means a major portion of what is necessary for well-being and life satisfaction is being neglected.

EMOTIONS RUN DEEP, BUT LIE HIDDEN

The subject of sexuality for people with disabilities has, until fairly recently, been generally taboo. Forced sterilization of individuals with some disabilities, such as cerebral palsy, was still being performed in the early 1960's in various states. In actuality, people with disabilities have been given the strong message to hold in check most of their feelings, especially anger, frustration, and sadness. Today's adults with cerebral palsy were often isolated and dependent on their parents as children; as a result, many have developed a habitually docile and complacent demeanor.

Most people with disabilities are implicitly or explicitly encouraged to avoid the negative emotional sides of their lives. This may be especially true for those with spinal cord injuries while in acute rehabilitation. The young man injured in an automobile or motorcycle accident, or by a gunshot wound or a sports injury, likely has a great deal of anger over the injury, its cause, and its often unavoidable consequences. To allow the expression of strong anger is to risk violent outbursts. Unvented anger, however, can manifest itself as depression, illness, and/or resistance to rehabilitation. A typical course of action is to glorify courage and toughness by idealizing others who exhibit these characteristics.

Ken, 1988 Continued

Fifteen years after his injury, Ken shared his perspective on the emotional aspects of rehabilitation. (The book that he mentions, *Options*, published by the National Spinal Cord Injury Association, is one that was circulated on his spinal cord injury hospital floor in 1974. It contains case examples of people's lives after their injuries and is meant to be inspiring.)

What's needed is a good middle ground between the attitude expressed in the book, *Options*, where you feel like a failure because you know you'll never match up to the guys in that book — who all have a $200,000-a-year job, a wife and kids, a big house and a brand new sports car — and the need to have some hope held out to you, which *Options* does to an extreme and which can destroy a lot of people attitudinally. Initially in rehabilitation you need a ray of hope. It gives you something to work toward. But professionals should be more realistic by telling people that, "This is possible, but not likely for everyone." As rehab moves along, they should emphasize more and more each person's own capabilities and what is realistic for that person. They also need to get people to see that their disability doesn't need to stand in the way of their achievement. You're going to have failures, but you're also going to have successes. Without trying, you're not going to have either.

I wasn't assertive before my injury, and that helped because the more aggressive guys with a lot of hostility and intolerance have a tougher time with their injuries.

Some people just need more time than others. There were people up on the floor that hated going to therapy. There was no motivation there whatsoever. So, for them, maybe therapy wasn't the answer at that point. They were the ones that got left by the wayside. The people that would come into their sessions and do what was expected, the staff seemed to concentrate more on them.

Some rehab professionals try to make silk purses out of sows' ears, and that isn't being realistic either. Rehab needs to have the attitude of, "Okay, this is what you have, and this is what you can work with. What can you do to make the best out of what you can work with?" They need to focus mainly on those people that are going day-to-day through life, just like the average non-disabled person goes day-to-day through life.

Ken's perspective was formed after a slow recovery from depression and prolonged rehabilitation, which he likened to Elisabeth Kubler-Ross's stages of dying (1969).

If someone is stuck in the grieving process... six to seven years is the average for real adjustment. It's like an adjustment to a death. The only thing is, for an injury or disability, it's not as easy to adjust as with a death because with a death, the person's no longer there. With a disability, you have a constant reminder. So, sometimes it takes even longer to grieve and adjust. A lot of people turn to alcohol and drugs, which is a way of going through denial. As long as you're smashed or stoned, you can forget about your disability. It alters the mind and you can forget about it. Well, you don't forget about it — you just don't quite care as much.

I asked Ken for his opinion about how common it is for people with spinal cord injuries to use drugs and alcohol to avoid confronting the facts of their disabilities. He continued,

Everybody goes through that stage, I think, of using a lot of alcohol or drugs. It's just a coping mechanism. Some break out of it and some don't. I know people who've stayed smashed their whole lives. If you use it just for a while, it's a good coping mechanism. You're usually left alone by society because when they see somebody with a disability, and see they're an alcoholic, they say, "Well, they've got enough problems. Let them be." Even in rehab, we used to be able to drink all we wanted. The hospital even supplied it. Just as long as you'd do rehab the next day, it was okay. I don't know exactly why. I think maybe because the doctors knew that no matter what they did for us, it was still inadequate. But now that policy has changed because they had too many problems with people getting really smashed and getting into fights. And one nurse's aide on drugs snapped out. I believe you can still get a couple of beers, but not as much as you used to be able to get.

Rohe and DePompolo (1985) reported the results of a survey of rehabilitation unit personnel on their substance abuse policies which indicate both that substance abuse at that time was quite prevalent and that the policies on Ken's rehabilitation unit were not uncommon, nor Ken's hunches inaccurate. (See also Heinemann, 1991; Benshoff, Janikowski, Taricone, & Brenner, 1990; Greer, 1986.) Current policies on most rehabilitation units in the U.S. have since changed to prohibit the use of alcohol and tobacco while on the unit, but a survey of staff at one facility indicates efforts to assess and treat these dependencies remains poor (Basford, Rohe & DePompolo 2003).

Ken summarized his perspective on adjustment for the person with a spinal cord injury as follows: "A lot of it is just time. Rehab can't turn your life around in just a couple of months." Many people with disabilities need time to develop an awareness of their disability and to achieve a perspective of themselves which allows them to admit grief and anger and then get on with their lives. Some need months; others need years. For Ken, it took a major life event to turn himself around.

> It was a slow process getting fed up with doing nothing. It was like a long, low-grade depression I didn't even know I had until I came out of it. It was just, I was unmotivated. I knew it even while I was doing it. But even when I was in the stage of depression or whatever, in the rut stage, I saw both the positive and negative sides. I never had a real negative attitude. I was in the stoned part, but I wasn't negative. I always tried to keep an optimistic attitude. I think that's what helped me to get out of the depression and progress through the stages.
>
> One of the things that did it, also, was not something I was glad happened, and that was my mother's death. My mother, and all my family, were very overprotective — but especially my mother. After she was gone, there was not so much of a dominant figure, so then I had to kind of learn to find my own way. My father... he was a very passive person, a farmer most of his life. He died two years ago and he kind of took things as they came and just went through life. Good or bad, I modeled him in a lot of ways... Even though I went through the depression and stuff, there's not a lot of ways to change things. You change things when you can, but you don't go out and constantly knock your head against a wall to try to beat down the system and this type of thing. You make little changes where you can in a... quieter way. And it does work. Once you can achieve smaller goals, you can work up.

Ken's example underscores the importance of on-going assessment for treating depression in persons with SCI. The prevalence of depression in persons with SCI is 25%-40% with less than 10% receiving a diagnosis and adequate treatment, in many cases due to the attitude, "If you have a spinal cord injury, you ought to be depressed" (Krause, Crewe & Kemp, 1999). Depressed persons have been shown to have lower ratings of overall health, life satisfaction and purpose in life (Cushman & Scherer, 1998; Krause, 1999).

Symptoms of Depression[1]
When someone is depressed, that person has several symptoms nearly every day, all day, that last at least 2 weeks. These symptoms include:

- Loss of interest in enjoyable activities, including sex*
- Feeling sad, blue, or down in the dumps*
- Feeling slowed down or feeling restless and unable to sit still
- Feeling worthless
- Changes in appetite or weight loss or gain
- Thoughts of death or suicide; suicide attempts
- Problems concentrating, thinking, remembering, or making decisions
- Trouble sleeping or sleeping too much
- Loss of energy or feeling tired all of the time

Other symptoms may include:
- Headaches
- Other aches and pains
- Digestive problems
- Sexual problems
- Feelings of pessimism or hopelessness
- Being anxious or worried

If a person has experienced five or more of these symptoms including at least one of the first two symptoms marked with an asterisk (*) for at least 2 weeks, they should tell their health care provider immediately. The successful treatment of depression today combines new drug treatments with psychotherapy for learning new problem-solving techniques and coping strategies.

Ken also made some good points regarding motivation. He talked first about a "psychological readiness" for rehabilitation ("Some people just need more time than others"), and then about the importance of achieving smaller goals "and then you can work up." This point was very similar to what Chris said in Chapter Four: "It's not just motivation, it takes a willingness on their part to work. They need to like a challenge... It's like, 'I won this little battle,' and it builds you up." But some people may never develop a motivation to get on with their lives, as Ken then noted:

> Through my years I've seen both sides of it. I mean, I've been in rehab so many times they don't want to see me again! But I've seen everything from really high achievers to suicides, you know, people that are planning suicide. Or a couple of people that I know of that are drinking themselves to death. It's just that different people look at it in somewhat different ways.

People with spinal cord injuries, particularly those with recent injuries, often have vacillating motivation during rehabilitation. Even years after their injury, it can still be difficult to sustain motivation. They often describe a kind of one-step-forward-two-back experience when starting a new job or returning to school. Those who "push their up time" on a regular basis can develop pressure sores which require hospitalization and an interruption in their activities. Steady forward progress in their lives is a challenge to achieve.

To illustrate: Ken started a graduate program in rehabilitation counseling in a city sixty miles from where he lives. He called me in the middle of the Fall 1991 semester to say we needed to postpone our get-together because he was trying to stop the growth of a pressure sore he had developed a couple of weeks before. His doctor told him that as soon as the sore got worse, he would have to stop his commuting. Now that the sore had gotten worse, he was reluctantly in the process of trying to arrange a medical leave from school. He did not want to do this, as it would mean taking an "incomplete" in a prerequisite for a Spring course. In essence, he was now faced with being a year behind schedule in his graduate program.

If such setbacks happen often to a person with marginal coping skills, they can reduce motivation and engender an increase in depression, withdrawal, and the development of a general negative outlook.

WAYS OF ADJUSTING TO DISABILITY CAN AND DO DIFFER

As with *rehabilitation success* and the *disability experience*, adjustment is dynamic, situational, and often "in the eye of the beholder." People vary as much in *how* they adjust to and cope with physical injury and permanent disability as they vary in the extent to which they do adjust and cope. One person may perform well at work, but not with the situation at home. As the situation improves at home, stressful new challenges may develop at work. A person may even report that he is doing well in all aspects of life, only to be told otherwise by rehabilitation professionals, employers, or family members.

As is true for people in general, some individuals with disabilities live with their challenges better than others. Some pursue a productive and satisfying life, others are "just sitting'" for a time, and still others seem destined to have their efforts to achieve a particular lifestyle repeatedly frustrated.

Brian said in 1986, "If I come across something that needs to be done, or that hinders me in any way, then I'll find a way that'll work." Butch, on the other hand, tended to give in to the obstacles posed by his spinal cord injury: "... now here I'm sittin'. Now there's no fightin' to come back." Some individuals with spinal cord injuries will harbor hopes for a cure and refuse to develop career or lifestyle plans compatible with their present capabilities. Some (like Ken and Brian) share an unwillingness to be held back from pursuing their independence and goals. Others seem to lack motivation for increasing their independence.

Hope is multidimensional and a powerful source of motivation. Some individuals have lost hope, some have hopes that can be viewed as unrealistic, and some have hopes that provide them with the confidence, purpose and meaning to participate fully in their rehabilitation. Hope can originate from many sources including faith and spirituality and medical and technological advances. While it is important to realize that unrealistic hopes, dreams and expectations (those without the means to achieve them) can be frustrating and disappointing, keeping dreams alive can result in an open mind to change and the exploration of options.

Research has shown a positive effect of spirituality in adjusting to a traumatic disability (McColl, Bickenbach, Johnston, Nishihama, Schumaker, Smith, Smith & Yealand, 2000). Some of these effects include a new understanding of trusting others, a greater awareness of the self and a sense of purpose in life that was not there before. These effects can in turn alter one's temperament and personality. Contrary to the belief that our personalities are well formed by middle adulthood, and are stable, a growing body of literature discusses both personality change and stability as occurring throughout our lives. Maslow viewed middle age as an opportunity for positive change. Erikson saw personality development as occurring over the lifespan. Susan Krauss Whitbourne's (2004) model of adult identity views identity development as a process in which people continually confirm or revise their self- perceptions based on experience and feedback from others. That is, we continue to revise and modify our identities and self-concept based upon our social exposures and experiences. Several participants reported having confused or fragile identities and feelings of being alienated from the rehabilitation system and from their peers who either do or do not have disabilities. While many emphasize their goals, their desire to work around obstacles, and the value of their assistive technologies, others focus on obstacles as being insurmountable. Some present themselves as meeting challenges head-on, others as feeling defeated.

All individuals showed variability in their emotional and psychological situations over time which reflected changes in both their adjustment and their circumstances. For example, Brian and Ann and Linda increasingly gained self-confidence. Jim did not, however, and consequently became "physically run down." Maggie's changed condition brought ups and downs in her life satisfaction. Such results demonstrate that people with disabilities adjust in various ways over time, that time may work to help their efforts or may set them back (e.g., with physical complications), and that psychological factors are important in the understanding of short- and long-term adjustment.

While an individual's background, experiences, beliefs, and personality play key roles in the definition of his or her *disability experience*, another influence is the type of motivation used by the person's family and rehabilitation team. Ken used the example of the individuals portrayed in the book, *Options*, as a particular type of motivator.

> It's one thing to give a ray of hope, everybody needs that; but it's quite another to indicate they can get up and walk again someday. They should build confidence without building hopes so high that people expect they can be completely normal. Assistive devices can help you, but they're not going to enable you to walk or to get back the use of your hands.... A lot of it is just time.

As important as allowing for the passage of time is looking beyond the physical aspects of rehabilitation to the psychosocial needs and quality of life of the person.

There is perhaps no better example of the variability that can occur in an individual's emotional and psychological state than Butch's experience.

Butch, 1991

Approaching Butch's house once again, I no longer had any feelings of apprehension or anxiety. This time I noticed food scattered in one area of the driveway for the squirrels and birds, and the van was sitting in a different part of the driveway than usual. As I was getting out of the car, a door opened and Butch's mother gestured for me to come in. Her warm greeting was followed by a few minutes of friendly conversation. Then I got on the elevator to take myself up to Butch's annex.

Once at the door, Butch responded to my knock with his booming but cheerful "C'mon in." Upon entering, I was shocked to come face-to-face with the biggest stuffed buffalo head I had ever seen. Butch, eclipsed by the thing and chuckling, peered out from around it and proceeded to tell me just how he had come to own this furry masterpiece. Then he pointed out his other recent acquisitions: a bearskin rug, a ram's head, and a five foot carved wooden bear. These were nothing, however, compared to the 10 x 6?-foot latch-hooked rug on the wall over the sofa. It portrayed The Last Supper; Butch had created it in just 57 days as a Christmas present for his mother.

Butch's life is now a busy one. He is nearing the end of the process of making a new power wheelchair. "I got together all the parts, welded them, and am doing the whole thing myself."

He goes out quite frequently. "There isn't a mall in the area I don't have memorized." He travels around primarily with family, but has a friend with whom he double-dated this past summer to go to a rock concert — his first ever. He does not yet dine out, however, since "I go into terrible spasms after I eat and who wants to see that?"

Overall, Butch says, "I enjoy myself more now. You know, it's been 3,328 days since my injury and it just got boring sitting here doing nothin'."

3,328 days — and counting.

Coping and Non-Coping

In Beatrice Wright's classic text, *Physical Disability: A Psychological Approach* (1960), considerable attention is devoted to coping and non-coping, which are defined as follows:

- *Coping* — [Seeing] the difficulties associated with a disability as something that [can] be faced in some way or overcome ... [focusing] on the adjustable aspects... coping with the difficulties rather than managing because of blissful ignorance or pretense (p. 59).

- *Succumbing (non-coping)* — [Seeing] difficulties as a quagmire through which there [is] no path. Perhaps one doesn't even seek a path, for one is so consumed with the suffering of the disabled state that one is dragged down by despair (p. 59).

In keeping with Wright, people who *cope* emphasize what they can do and seek to satisfy achievement and affiliation needs; persons who *succumb* focus on what they cannot do. People who *cope* pursue opportunities; people who *succumb* are more passive, downplay their competence and do not strive to enhance it, and distrust the opportunities presented to them. *Coping* behaviors are employed to overcome limitations — through further education, the development of new skills, and the use of assistive technologies; *succumbing* is characterized by a resignation to and a concentration on limitations.

Cycles of Hope and Despair

Coping, adjustment and the achievement of a personally satisfying quality of life, involve achieving or maintaining control. When a person experiences a severe trauma, such as a spinal cord injury, a major disequilibrium occurs. This may occur on a family level as well as for the individual with the new disability. Some individuals with recently acquired disabilities may not have had earlier experiences and exposures essential to the development of successful decision-making, responsibility, and self-control. Individuals born with cerebral palsy were rarely given such opportunities. Therefore, a new or additional disability, deteriorating health, a change in one's family or financial situation, can overtax a person's psychological resources. While crises are difficult for anyone to handle, they can be especially so for persons with disabilities who have not had opportunities for learning and practicing ways to manage a variety of situations.

Robert Sternberg, a past president of the American Psychological Association has said,

"...what distinguishes those who are highly successful from others, in large part, resilience in the face of humiliation, defeats and setbacks of various kinds. For those who do not have some kind of optimism... it often seems much easier just to start watching the world go by instead of actively participating in it" (p.5).

Humiliation, defeats and setbacks affect each and every one of us; no one is immune from them. Thus, the issue is not avoiding them, because that is impossible. The key to success is coming out of them with optimism, dreams, and goals.

Coping and adjustment can vary between phenomenal success and marginal success. Non-coping, too, varies from complete and continued withdrawal, helplessness, and hopelessness to maintaining marginal functioning that may develop over time into coping and adjustment. As we develop and mature, we formulate new strategies for goal achievement. When they work and we are successful, it appears we are coping. Should our strategies fail us for a time, we may exhibit non-coping behaviors. Coping and non-coping people display significant differences that vary according to the settings in which they find themselves and the kind and amount of personal, professional, social and financial resources available to them.

As we saw in Jim's case, one may experience "phenomenal success" at one point in time and marginal coping, or even succumbing, at another. Or one may cope with some life situations better than others.

Examples abound of persons who appear to be *succumbing* and later manifest *coping*. In 1986, Butch appeared to be succumbing. Yet anyone familiar with persons with disabilities knows that a random sample will reflect as wide a range of diversity as is found in the population as a whole. There will be pessimists and optimists, religious and nonreligious individuals, Type A personalities and passive people, angry people and easygoing people, people with a good social support network and people in social conflict, people who are denying the facts of their disability, people who have actively sought out all the information they can about their disability, and so on. It is impossible to look at the personality of each of these individuals and accurately predict who will be a future rehabilitation success and who will not. To think there is conclusive evidence for predictable emotional and mental patterns in coping and adjustment is to do a tremendous disservice to all persons who have a disability.

Still, succumbing to a lifestyle of dependence is certainly a different personal statement from a spirited determination and drive to overcome obstacles to achievement and independence. To help a person move from withdrawal and hopelessness to adjustment and coping requires attention to physical, social, developmental, and psychological/personal factors, but in a studied and cautious manner. To omit the effects of time and of individuals' attempts to think about and understand their disability and act on their own behalf ignores the positive growth principle implied in Maslow's hierarchy.

SUMMARY

Figure 7-3 summarizes the discussion up to now. A person with a particular disability will experience physical, psychological, and psychosocial consequences of that disability, which in turn create that individual's *disability experience*, personal definition of rehabilitation success, and expectations regarding *quality of life*. These factors will then determine features of the milieu/environment, person, and assistive technology (AT) which predispose the individual to AT use or non-use. The person will ultimately use or not use a particular AT. Now the direction reverses: Non-use, or successful/satisfying use, of an AT will further impact the person, the person's milieu, and the recommendation of additional devices. These developments will lead the individual to reexamine her view of *rehabilitation success*, the *disability experience* and *quality of life* and will affect the person physically, psychologically and socially.

Because these concepts are subjective, multi-dimensional, interactive and individualized, they are also difficult to define. That is why the substance of the next chapter is a concept-by-concept description of a model designed to identify facilitators of (and, conversely, barriers to) a person's use of a particular technology.

The dynamic interactive relationship among AT use, quality of life, functional capabilities, preferences, and so on, requires a person-

Figure 7-3: Assistive Technology (AT) Use as Both an Influence On and an Outcome of "Disablility"

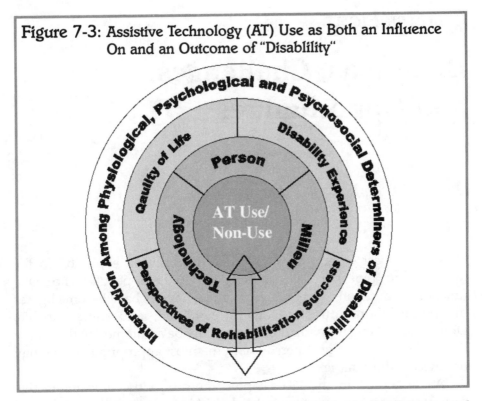

centered focus on the achievement of need satisfaction and "essential attachments" in light of limitations in physical functioning. Achieving the best possible match of person and technology is now a key element of individual need satisfaction; therefore, it must become a crucial component of the rehabilitation process.

Footnotes Chapter Seven

[1]Adapted from: Agency for Health Care Policy and Research (AHCPR). (1993, April). *Depression Is A Treatable Illness: A Patient's Guide*. Washington, DC: Author. AHCPR Publication No. 93-0553.

CHAPTER EIGHT

Dilemmas, Challenges, and Opportunities

Why, then the world's mine oyster,
Which I with sword will open.
— **SHAKESPEARE**

During the past several decades, there has been an explosion in the number and types of devices designed to help people who have functional limitations. Over the years, these devices have become lighter in weight, more attractive and streamlined, and more flexible. Differences among individual users can now be accommodated, making the process of matching a person with the most appropriate technology or device quite complex.

As discussed in the last chapter, there is a dynamic interactive relationship among assistive technology (AT) use, quality of life, and the user's functional capabilities and temperament. Therefore, the complexity of matching an individual with the most appropriate AT demands a person-centered focus. To ensure use of the device(s), there must also be a social climate which values enhanced functional capability, and a psychological readiness and motivation for AT use on the part of the individual with a disability and, if relevant, their caregivers.

While millions of people use assistive technology devices, many others discard or abandon them. Studies show rates of abandonment ranging from 8% to 75%, depending on the type of device. On average, about one-third of all devices are abandoned. We have no information about the numbers of people who continue to use devices they are unhappy or uncomfortable with because they cannot abandon them without facing more severe consequences.

Most abandonment occurs either within the first year (especially the first three months) or after five years of use (the elapsed time before Medicaid or Medicare insurance will fund a replacement). These statistics suggest that users learn relatively quickly whether a device works for them. If it doesn't, it is quickly discarded. If it does, the user may keep it until it needs to be replaced — usually after five or more years.

The non-use of recommended technology can have a series of repercussions such as decreases in functional abilities, loss of freedom and independence, increases in expenses, and risk of injury or disease. Device abandonment also represents ineffective use of limited funds by federal, state, and local government agencies, insurers, and other providers. A better understanding of how and why technology users decide to accept or reject a device is critical to improving the effectiveness of assistive technology devices and services, and to enhancing consumer satisfaction with them.

The single most significant factor associated with technology abandonment is a failure to consider the user's opinions and preferences in device selection — in other words, *the device is abandoned because it does not meet the person's needs or expectations*. Phillips and Zhao (1993) list other major reasons (in no particular order):

- lack of motivation to use the device or do the task for which the device is intended

- changes in the user's functional abilities or activities requiring new, upgraded functions which the device cannot accommodate

- lack of meaningful training on how to use the device (especially for elderly or cognitively impaired individuals) and/or lack of ongoing rehabilitation team support

- ineffective device performance

- accessibility problems

- lack of access to and information about repair and maintenance

- the device was unnecessary; the person needs a more comprehensive intervention

- the device is so complicated it confuses the user and overtaxes care givers

Most of these issues can be addressed appropriately in a *comprehensive* evaluation and selection process that considers the person's ongoing needs, takes a long-term view of an individual's assistive device use, and is, first and foremost, focused on the user's interests, needs, readiness, and capabilities. It is important to have a concrete plan and reason for the use of a device which takes into account potential future needs. Finally, training the user (and others who support and/or live with the user) for device use should be done in the settings in which it will be used, focusing on how the device can best be used in those environments.

MATCHING A PERSON WITH THE MOST APPROPRIATE TECHNOLOGY

The desire for — and reactions to — assistive technologies are highly individual. Ultimately, the goal of rehabilitation professionals is to match an individual with an assistive device that will enhance the person's capabilities and quality of life. Regardless of the type of device, an individual will either use it or not use it, to varying degrees. Non-use can consist of device abandonment, or avoidance of a device altogether (e.g., a person will not show up for an evaluation or fitting or will not purchase it). Use can be full-time and done willingly, or partial and done inappropriately or reluctantly. Partial use most frequently occurs when users:

a. experience fatigue or discomfort when using the device,

b. have other options than the device, or

c. use a device in one setting but not another.

Need Determines Use

We know that the highest rate of assistive technology use occurs when an individual's functioning is highly limited, when viable alternatives to use do not exist, are not available, or are less desirable, or when a person experiences clear gains from use. For example, everyone mentioned in this book uses a wheelchair; the only alternative for them would be a lack of mobility. A person with cerebral palsy who has little or no intelligible speech will be a more frequent user of a communication device than someone who has difficulty with only certain words. Thus, the *degree to which an assistive device is essential for desired functioning* influences its use. As a former director of a rehabilitation unit said to me,

> It seems the more the device is needed for self-care and independence both in and outside of the home, the more it is used. A classic example involves almost 100% prosthetic arm use by someone without any arms, but if one arm is normal, use falls drastically.

According to another rehabilitation professional,

> [Non-use of communication devices] is due in part to the fact that communication is a very fast process and no current device provides the same speed — although some are getting close. It depends on the person and what that person wants to say and how adept she or he is at saying it.

Figure 8-1: Influences on Assistive Technology Use*

		Milieu	Person	Technology
U S E	**Optimal**	• Information available about options • User involved in device selection • Support from family/peers/employer • Realistic expectations of family/employer • Setting/environment supports and encourages use	• Realistic expectations of device • Motivated for device use • Cooperative • Optimistic • Self-determining • Good decision-making skills • Self-advocating • Patient and self-disciplined • Positive life experiences and mood • Has the skills for device use • Perceives discrepancy between desired and current situation (wants more autonomy)	• Achieves goal without pain, fatigue or stress • Compatible with/enhances the use of other supports • Is safe, reliable, easy to use and maintain • Has the desired transportability • No better options currently available • Adequate preparation for use and training
	Partial/ Reluctant/ Inappropriate	• Pressure for use (therapist, family, peers, employer) • Support often not available • Setting/ environment discourages use or makes use difficult or uncomfortable	• Embarrassed to use device • Unmotivated to use device • Impatient/impulsive • Unrealistic expectations • Low self-esteem • Somewhat intimidated by technology • Device partially or occasionally fits with lifestyle • Deficits in skills needed for use • Lacks confidence in ability to use device	• Goal not fully achieved or with discomfort/strain • Requires a lot of set-up • Interferes somewhat with the use of other supports • Interferes with normal routines and customary ways of doing things • Device is inefficient • Better options exist • Feelings of insecurity with use • Little or no training provided for use • Other changes, not AT, were needed

Figure 8-2: Influences on Assistive Technology Use*

		Milieu	Person	Technology
N O N U S E	**Avoidance**	• Lack of support for use from family/peers/employer • Unrealistic expectations of others • Funding not available • Setting/environment disallows or prevents use • Culture devalues use	• Embarassed to use device • Depressed • Not motivated, resistant to change • Uncooperative • Withdrawn • Not comfortable with technology • Use requires unwanted changes in lifestyle • Negative outlook • Does not have skills for use • Prefers help from others	• Unsatisfactory prior device use • Benefit not apparent • Too much strain or discomfort in use • Requires a lot of set-up • Incompatible with the use of other supports • Too expensive • Long delay for delivery • Alternatives seen as preferable (e.g., personal assistance)
	Abandonment/ Discard	• Lack of support for use from family/peers/employer • Setting/environment discourages use or makes use difficult or uncomfortable • Requires support that is not available • Device choice made only by therapist • Need for upgrades not assessed	• Unrealistic expectations of benefit • Embarrassed or self-conscious about using device • Depressed • Low self-esteem • Hostile/angry • Withdrawn • Resistant • Many changes in lifestyle with device use • Lacks skills to use device and training is not available	• Goal not achieved • Did not match goals or expectations • Discomfort/strain in use • Is incompatible with the use of other supports • Has been outgrown • Is difficult to use • Device is inefficient • Repairs/service not timely or affordable • Other and preferred options became available • Additional limitations preclude use

*These points summarize much of the discussion and literature regarding the use of AT. Additional summary points associated with less than optimal technology use is a failure to consider the user's opinions and preferences in device selection — in other words, *the individual's needs, preferences and expectations were not adequately or thoroughly assessed*. Only during such an assessment can the rehabilitation professional make the best judgment regarding the impact of:
• Related limitations (such as low vision)
• Outlook, adjustment, attitude and mood
A thorough assessment is also needed to adequately address:
• Functional *capabilities* as well as limitations
• Need for an AT (and equipping the person) versus modifying the environment or the family's responses and support
• Level of need for training and identification of settings for trial use (home, work, school)

I know if I had to spell out every word I wanted to say, especially after having a normal rate of speech, I'm not going to say very much and I'm not going to use very long sentences. With a device, communication comes across as terse and all sorts of subtleties are lost.

As the example of Chuck showed in Chapter One, individuals with severe disabilities require not only more equipment, but more expensive equipment.

The Desirability of a Model for Matching Person and Technology

The factors that influence the use or non-use of more optional assistive technologies (not essential to the user) can be viewed as follows:

1. The characteristics of the **Milieu** or setting(s) in which the assistive technology is to be used.

2. The pertinent features of the individual's **Personality**, temperament, and preferences.

3. The salient characteristics of the assistive **Technology** itself.

Matching people with the most appropriate assistive technology for them involves the consideration of many factors and influences within the above three domains. The "Matching Person and Technology (MPT)" model (Scherer, 1998) was first developed in 1989 to organize these influences and a portion is shown in Figure 8-1.

Considering these factors provides both a broad and an in-depth profile of where persons may be at a particular point in time with their devices. For example, a person may look like a partial or reluctant device user as far as the *milieu factors*, but appear to be an optimal user according to the characteristics listed for *personality and technology*. Thus, the *milieu* in which the device will be used may need some modification so the person can derive maximal satisfaction and functional gain from the device.

Assistive device use is interactive; changes in one set of factors will have an effect on the others. For example, optimal use of one assistive device may likely lead to enthusiasm for trying another device, improved self-confidence, and perhaps, a broadening of one's social community. It is also true that a person can use one device well and have qualms about using a second device at the same time. Sometimes, the introduction of a new device can make the use of an existing one more complicated or cumbersome. It is likely that as time goes on, device compatibility or incompatibility will be a growing area of concern. We are learning that a threshold can be reached when a system requiring management of multiple devices has an additive effect, resulting in frustration and overload for a person, and even such difficulties as repetitive motion injuries.

An assessment process emerged from the Matching Person and Technology model which consists of checklist-type instruments to record consumer goals and preferences, views of the benefits to be gained from a technology, and changes in self-perceived outcome achievement over time. The instruments are described in Appendix D. One set of instruments, the *Assistive Technology Device Predisposition Assessment* (ATD PA), was developed by studying differences between assistive technology users and non-users. It inquires into individuals' subjective satisfaction with current functioning in many areas and where the most improvement is desired. The consumer version has two forms: a) questions given per consumer on capabilities, subjective well-being, temperament and psychosocial resources and b) questions per technology on the consumer's views of and expectations for using that particular technology. Companion professional forms exist so that comparisons of professional and consumer views can be made. Data on reliability and validity to date indicate that they are quality assessments (Scherer & Craddock, 1998; Crewe and Dijkers, 1995). Appendix D provides sample items from the ATD PA as well as an example of a report discussing the results gained from using it. As you read the following sections in this chapter, you will note how the report addresses many of the points and issues discussed.

Characteristics of the Milieu

The environments in which the person uses a device or technology will either support or discourage use. As shown in Figure 8-1, relevant features of the milieu extend beyond physical access, often requiring social and economic support.

Consumers of assistive technology services include persons with disabilities (primary consumers) and their family members and caregivers (secondary consumers). It is important to involve all people who will be affected by the assistive technology at the outset, keeping in mind the function to which the technology will be put and the environment(s) in which it will operate and be used. According to one rehabilitation engineer,

> The crucial step is to have the individual try it, to go through the routine of actually using the equipment or mimicking the use of that equipment. Usually with a device comes a need for extra room. If the individual is not able to use it you can look for other alternatives, see if there's need for

further modification, etc. Sometimes you may have to start all over again. It's a man–machine interface where you're trying to get that individual with that particular disability able to operate a device in one or more environments. Many times I feel more like a social worker. You become an investigator, a detective. You find out what the different alternatives are within the constraints.

The value of offering trial periods before finalizing a technology selection cannot be overstated. The consumer must try the device in the actual situations of use (home, work, school).

Sometimes, even though an assistive device is requested, what is really needed is an environmental modification, or changes in the family's responses and support. Removing carpeting and steps, replacing or rearranging furniture, or adjusting the height of outlets, appliances, and countertops are examples of modifications that can eliminate the need for an assistive device or make a less expensive, low-tech option workable.

One of the most common reasons for the non-use or reluctant use of an assistive technology is that it was forced upon the person by family members or therapists. This is very common with children. Just as some families will resist the use of technological assistance, many will purchase anything they believe will help their child, only to discover that the child either does not want to use it or cannot use it.

Primary and secondary consumers need to have information about the advantages of a technology and know why, when, and under what circumstances it will be most useful.

Exposure and opportunity. Factors such as environmental accommodations, available resources (e.g., private insurance which covers devices, or availability of personal assistance), and special opportunities (e.g., placement in a rehabilitation center with the newest equipment) are also important milieu characteristics. Often, however, rehabilitation can seem like a "one-shot chance" to consumers, as expressed by Chuck:

I wish it was set up so that you could go home for a year and then come back. Just so you could get more work done in some areas and strengthen points you want to work on, and where you'd have a therapist who would give you ideas on how to make things better at home. I mean, don't go just cold turkey. Usually once you're done with rehab, that's it, you're done with rehab.... But it would be great to have that individual help after a year or so.

Prior experiences and expectations, particularly for those with congenital disabilities, play an important role, as one rehabilitation professional describes:

> Many of our people with cerebral palsy always had someone to take care of them. They never had to cope with things and they haven't developed those skills, they never learned them. Also, they tend to have low opinions of their abilities — "I can't feed myself," "I can't do the simplest things other people take for granted." To be a successful user of a device requires patience and perseverance. Suffocating families and institutions sap individuals of enthusiasm, the hope that something new and exciting can still happen. When you see an assistive device as an opportunity to better your life and situation, then you're willing to pay the price of a long, tiring, frustrating trial-and-error period of learning. If the desire and perseverance aren't there, the frustration is too great — and after a short trial the device is shoved in the closet because it was too much of a hassle or it was just too overwhelming.

Some of the most frequent problems encountered by persons with cerebral palsy in the use of communication devices include the individual's lack of such fundamental communication skills as topic initiation and conversational turn-taking (Creech, 1990; Bjorck-Akesson, 1990; Musselwhite, 1990). Unless users have the opportunity to use and practice these skills, their device use will not be optimal.

A peer user of the same or a similar device can provide tremendous support and assistance during the trial period of device use.

Expectations Held By Others. The attitudes of others and their expectations of the consumer can have a profound influence on persons with disabilities and their expectations of themselves. What may seem to be a vital task to one person may be of small value to another. The self-concept, motivation, and personal aspirations of an individual are shaped by resources, opportunities, and supportive social interactions.

An equally important influence on a person's achievement of a rehabilitation goal is the character of the goal itself — specifically, to maximize the chance it will be achieved, the goal should be (a) explicit, (b) close to where the person's performance currently is, and (c) not too difficult. An additional influence, of course, is reinforcing the experience of success accompanying the process towards goal achievement.

> For new users especially, it is helpful to take things one step at a time, rewarding each accomplishment.

Social support. It is important to distinguish persons who report being *lonely* from those who are *isolated*. *Loneliness* is a subjective sense of being alone, even when surrounded by significant others; *isolation*, on the other hand, implies a dearth of social contacts. Loneliness requires a more psychological intervention, whereas isolation suggests a need for increased social opportunities which may be greatly facilitated by assistive technology use.

An acquired disability often places sudden strains on family relationships and social resources. When the support network is altered, the person may experience both psychological and physical distress, which can lead to a further disorganization, deterioration, and disintegration of the social support system.

Assistive device users tend to have more social support than nonusers. For example, successful users had families who built ramps and modified the family home, or employers who held jobs open for them. Other factors that promoted successful technology use were the person's position as family wage-earner, the family's commitment to learn how to assist in the operation and maintenance of the assistive device(s), and the family's positive attitude from the outset toward the person's need for the assistive device(s).

> Asking the individual about his or her social and material support, including cultural preferences, is an important part of understanding the impact of milieu influences on use or non-use.

Culture. The individual's cultural identity and the values and norms of that culture should be considered. The conclusions drawn in a paper by Parette, Huer & Scherer (2004), are meant to help professionals discover more appropriate AT devices from a broader culturally sensitive perspective. For example, when using the *Matching Person and Technology* assessment forms with a Native American male having a C6 spinal cord injury, some accommodations needed to be made. While he liked the parts of the assessment focusing on positive aspects of life functioning, other components were more difficult since his past experiences with AT could not be expressed using his native language. Compounding the challenge was a strongly held Native American cultural value (i.e., minimization of self-disclosure to others) that inhibited his ability to discuss issues of a personal nature, particularly when the person asking questions was a female.   The intensity of the emotions exhibited by the interviewee during this assessment process, and the insights gained by the interviewer were marked:

> It was obvious that he wanted to answer accurately, but he struggled immensely with those items that he described as being weak in character. I told him that we did not have to complete this form if he was too uncomfortable. He stated that he was uncomfortable but also knew that his responses would be important. On several of his answers, he began to cry and we had to give him time to recover and talk about the emotion before moving on. At one point all four of the team members were in tears from the emotion that the consumer had shared with us. I struggled with the process of completing the surveys because I felt that they were violating a very private part of this consumer. I don't recall exactly when the revelation hit me, but I do remember the insight that I suddenly had - even though the consumer had experienced emotional pain during the process, it was an avenue that had allowed this Native American to release his feelings and talk about deep rooted issues that had been a part of him for years. It was actually cathartic in nature and was moving him from a place of despair to a place of hope. When I finally realized this, I understood the importance of the MPT process. It isn't just about finding the right assistive technology for a consumer, it is about a person-centered process that takes a consumer through a progression of steps to become more comfortable with his/her disability and more independent in all areas of his/her life (Parette, Huer & Scherer, 2004, p.36-7).

As the above quote indicates, acculturation (i.e., attitudinal and cultural factors) comprises a key component of a technology user's perspective of AT, support use in general, and degree of confidence and trust in professionals and their recommendations. Regional differences exist in predispositions to particular devices as well as therapist recommendations. Additionally, as pointed out by Thomason (1990), the physical environments of use vary among cultures. For example, before planning to equip rural Native Americans with assistive devices, he advises the consideration of such factors as terrain, the availability of electricity, etc.

Characteristics of the Person

Individuals who use assistive devices say they have goals they want to pursue, believe obstacles to their independence can be overcome, tend to focus on expanding their capabilities, have their eyes on opportunities rather than on limitations, and believe they control their quality of life. They often are dissatisfied with their current situation and see benefits to

AT use that they value. Device users are not easily discouraged; in fact, they enjoy challenge. If funding for a device proves challenging, they will find a way to get what they want. As noted by a former director of a rehabilitation unit who is now the director of a medical division for a large corporation:

> It appears that assistive device use depends on the person's decision that (1) he or she was going to perform a given task and (2) that it could not be done without a device. Often, time, learning, doing, and yearning is necessary before that decision is made. Systems (and people) which force the decision on the person prematurely are flawed.

Technical comfort. The assumption that all people with disabilities have the desire to effectively utilize a computer-operated device is not an accurate one. Women in our society who grew up with little exposure to technologies tend to be uninformed about computers and disinterested in the complex and sophisticated products of rehabilitation engineering efforts (Littrell, 1991; Scherer, 1991b, 1991c). Non-technically oriented males, on the other hand, can feel even more threatened by high-tech devices, since they may feel an additional assault to their egos because they lack traditionally male skills.

Persons without the education, socialization, or exposure to the use of complex technologies can exhibit anxiety when faced with them. Being anxious makes it more difficult for them to learn the skills required to operate a sophisticated device. In addition to feeling anxious around high-tech devices, people often have a distrust of them, which is frequently borne out by experience (such as a stalled power wheelchair; Ann and Linda, Chapter Six).

Enders (1984) notes that among the general population of persons with disabilities, there are individuals who are intimidated by high-tech assistive devices (technophobes), and there are those who want only high-tech devices (technophiles). If high-tech devices are forced on a technophobic person, the devices often end up being unused or abandoned. But, according to Enders, an equally nonproductive situation results if a technophile is given everything he or she requests. Then, the glitzy and innovative qualities may take precedence over the functional ones, and a device will only be used until the next new innovation comes along.

Typically, technophobic individuals are persons who have not been exposed to technologies or who have had unsuccessful experiences with them. For them, the potential of achieving limited gains through the use of an assistive device is not worth the expense, anxiety, or discomfort involved in its use. Some aging persons, for example, reject technologies because they prefer to save their money, or because they resist the idea that they need help, or because they do not want to be seen using a device associated with loss of function. As one rehabilitation professional notes, this situation will no doubt change as people become increasingly exposed to technologies at very young ages.

> Most children with disabilities today are exposed to computers at a fairly young age. So a computer to them is not like a strange box that they don't know how to operate. It's no more strange than their wheelchair or eyeglasses. For the people who are seeing their first computer at the age of fifty, and who managed for fifty years without it, the device doesn't make a significant enough difference to warrant all that effort to learn to use it. This is a transition time. In thirty years it will all be commonplace and everyone will have equipment.

Technophobia is not always associated with age and previous exposure to technologies. We can all think of teenagers who are not drawn to computer use and grandmothers who have learned to use a PC expertly. Unless there are benefits derived from the use of a technology — be it a computer, food processor or assistive device — above and beyond what is achievable through currently available options, it will not be used. Nor will it be used if it requires too many modifications in one's daily routines and interactions with others.

When a person feels anxious or self-conscious about the use of a device in public, his interactions with others can become more strained, especially since assistive devices signal a disability and often set a person apart as appearing different. As Chuck mentioned in Chapter One, assistive devices can both physically and socially separate persons with disabilities from those without disabilities. Since an individual's self-esteem and self-image are built up over time through interactions with others, the presence of assistive devices can define those interactions and ultimately the elements of a person's self-image. Having assistive technologies be as non-visible as possible is a goal shared by many persons with disabilities.

Cognitive skills. People differ in their aptitudes to effectively use assistive devices. If an individual cannot read or spell, then a computerized device that relies on reading or spelling as input would be inappropriate for that person without a good deal of remedial work or other training; non-verbal, pictorial devices may be preferable. If a device requires more than a two-step command, a person who does not understand or manage sequence well, who is highly distractible, or who has a very short memory span may be frustrated by that device. So might the person who has been given a device that requires the development of unusual or new skills or that requires a large amount of conscious effort to control it. As explained by one rehabilitation professional,

> It is not helpful to ask more of a person than he or she can realistically be expected to deliver. For example, a high school graduate with fourth-grade reading and math skills will not become a capable clerical person until he or she shows at least a seventh-grade ability. So I don't buy this person a word processor prematurely.

Unlike Maggie, many persons her age born with cerebral palsy lack the basic educational background to take advantage of the opportunities afforded them by technological advances, particularly computerized devices. The emphasis technology places on cognitive and perceptual capabilities, as opposed to motor and physical skills, has opened many opportunities for persons with physical disabilities but has created some barriers for persons with cognitive, perceptual or learning disabilities. For them, a multi-sensory approach to device training works best, since computer use involves the person's auditory, visual, and tactile senses. For those with mild limitations, it is also helpful to supply the user with memory aids such as cards listing the sequence of steps to follow in operating devices.

Personality and temperament. Many spinal-cord-injured persons accustomed to risk-taking and being adventuresome find it difficult to adapt to a computer's discipline, especially those who, as Chris put it, had been "more at home with their bodies than with their minds." On the other hand, people with cerebral palsy who have been socialized to be quiet and passive often adapt to the computer's structure easily and willingly.

Device use is more acceptable when options are available and the person can exercise choice over the selection of features. While a wheelchair is not usually an optional piece of equipment for a person, the type and number of wheelchairs a person has is under more individual control. Chuck has two wheelchairs, one for traveling outdoors and one he uses only inside the house. When Chris was working, she had a wheelchair at home and both a wheelchair and a scooter at work. But for many persons, it is not financially possible to have multiple wheelchairs. These persons may feel their options are restricted, as noted by one woman with cerebral palsy:

It would be nice if the [power wheelchair] could be folded up and put in the trunk of a car. More streamlined, smaller, not as heavy. I'd rather be able to use a manual chair. Vehicles are not adapted for electric chairs. Because I can't ride in many vehicles and need to be bodily carried in and out of cars, I get left out of a lot of things I'd like to do, things I'd like to do with my husband. I can't go to all the places he can. [Her husband uses a manual wheelchair].

Assistive technology use, however, usually requires the person to admit that he or she cannot, and possibly never will, do a particular functional task independently. It means admitting a loss or functional limitation, and this can be distressing. A push for premature device use can be a mistake for those individuals who, as Butch said, "first need time to get used to just the thought of it." Both Butch and Ken eventually "got fed up with doing nothing." For them, *boredom* was a motivator out of the state of stuck. Later, a desire for regained control and independence led them to enhanced assistive technology use.

Many individuals with disabilities harbor hopes for a cure for their disability, or say they are waiting for highly touted experimental devices which they see as superior to those currently available. Such hopes often serve to hinder their rehabilitation. They should be encouraged to use existing technologies until the "superior" ones become available.

Individuals who have low self esteem, who are unaccustomed to being assertive and who have a personality style that makes it difficult for them to self-advocate, can find themselves in a situation, as stated by Brian, where their "*stuckness* feeds on itself:"

A friend who's a quad has a chair that is completely broken. He doesn't have the insurance I have so he's been stuck for 3 weeks. But he's very passive about things. If that happened to me, I'd be on the phone every two minutes demanding they get over and fix my chair. He's stuck in more ways than one. He's a computer programmer and can't find a job, his self-esteem is so low he doesn't want to interact with anyone other than his very closest friends. He doesn't make the effort to branch out and make new friends. So one thing affects one thing that influences another and you end up stuck. Low esteem, not assertive, stuck at home, narrow circle of friends…. Stuckness feeds on itself. It's usually not one thing but a number of things coming together. A combination of a lot of things combined. Then the spark and energy is gone. You need to pick one and fix that, then move on to the next one. "

This is not a new observation or insight from Brian and is consistent with his words and his lifestyle since I first met him. Once again, Chris' statement comes to mind: "Once you've won one little battle, it builds you up."

Counseling may be indicated for those persons who are angry, depressed, have a low self-esteem or who have never mastered how to make successful choices. Providing users with information in advance increases their control; by knowing what is likely to occur, they can better prepare for the outcome.

Judgment and preference. Many persons prefer to use a personal assistant or what capabilities they themselves have, however limited, rather than a mechanical replacement for their limited functions. Consumers can also differ in their judgments of the potential functional gains assistive devices offer them, as the following quote from a speech-language therapist indicates.

One person with cerebral palsy, for example, may determine that a device will not improve her speech intelligibility enough to warrant its use, while another equally affected individual may see a device as not only desirable, but indispensable. I am working with a person now who found her own balance. She has made very effective use of a small, portable, communication device by using it to augment a word here and there.

Assistive technologies are used when consumers see the device as valuable to their goal achievement. When the user has significant input into device selection, he or she becomes more invested in using it successfully.

Adjustment and outlook. Different physical disabilities are associated with varying complications, and thus with various courses of treatment and rehabilitation. Even people with the same or similar disabilities will attach different meanings to what has happened to them and what their future is likely to hold. Pre-existing temperament and ways of coping are just two factors that can influence adjustment and the length and quality of the recovery and rehabilitation process.

An individual born with a disability may have incorporated the disability into his or her self-image and have accepted the disability and the lifestyle modifications it may require. Individuals with cerebral palsy often view assistive technologies as opening up new vistas and making available new experiences and opportunities. On the other hand, many persons experiencing a spinal cord injury in early adulthood, or a stroke in middle age, may view assistive technologies as reminders of the independent functioning they have lost. Their disabilities can represent a major life change requiring modification in the person's basic identity and established ways of doing things. This can be met with resentment, as Chuck indicated in Chapter One: "Your basic style doesn't change just because you're in a wheelchair and the only things you can move are from the neck up."

As Ken said, the process of adjustment to a spinal cord injury may include periods of depression and pessimism, during which a person has a negative outlook about his or her future. Persons with spinal cord injuries frequently take seven or more years to come to terms with their disabilities. Many refer to the drastic adjustments they must make by talking, as Brian does, in terms of their "two lives." Often the "second life" means one has adopted a different lifestyle and outlook. But, just as Brian has maintained his strong recreational interests, so too have many others with spinal cord injuries. Research by Rohe and Krause (1992) has shown that the occupational and recreational interests of 79 men with spinal cord injuries remained stable in spite of their injury. There was no decrease of interest in physically demanding and adventuresome activities.

Characteristics of the Assistive Technology

An assistive technology is abandoned or discarded when:

1. It does not improve functioning beyond what the person is currently using or alternatives that the individual judges as being better or easier.

2. Servicing and repair were difficult to obtain and/or were very expensive.

3. The device performed unreliably.

4. The person felt uncomfortable, insecure or embarrassed using it.

When the device itself was satisfactory, consumers often report that the abandonment or replacement of a device was caused by changes in their priorities or needs.

Often several trade-offs need to be kept in mind — for example, between the unattractiveness of a device and certain functional gains — and that an individual's long-term gains sometimes require short-term stress, e.g., the family initially will have to build a ramp and (re)arrange transportation.

Design factors. Assistive technologies with the highest rate of use are:
• lightweight and portable

- easy to use and set up
- compatible with other devices
- cost-effective to obtain and maintain
- safe and reliable
- attractive as well as durable
- the same as or similar to devices used by the non-disabled population

A shortfall in any of these categories discourages use, as does user frustration with a device's speed, size or complexity.

The flexibility of devices and the degree to which they can accommodate the addition of other devices are also important. The increased practice of integrating multiple devices so they can be controlled by a single input device may create a more streamlined appearance, but may also result in cognitive overload — operations become too complex to learn easily or to recall quickly. Device complexity is also why scalable devices that accommodate growth and development are often abandoned.

The expense of individualized/customized products (i.e., does what the person wants without extraneous features to add to complexity and breakdown) need to be weighed against less satisfactory low-cost alternatives. In summary, devices are unlikely to be used if they "never seem to be there when needed," are seen as "not worth all the effort," do not have enough practical applications, and create discomfort or inconvenience. When caretakers view devices as requiring too much work and effort, they will not use them:

> Another point parents make is that the machine is always in the wrong room. They move the child or the child moves around, and they go for the device and it's not there. "Oh well, forget it then."

A rehabilitation engineer gave his wish list for the design of assistive technologies in the future, which is compatible with the wishes of consumers reported earlier:

> Encourage the development of smaller, and not so cumbersome, models of the equipment. The portability and packaging, outer looks, of the device should be as aesthetically pleasing as possible. Devices should be non-visible. We should maximize the use of current components used in industry in order for non-disabled people to be able to identify with device users more. I also want to highlight the need for streamlining designs to try to make them "acceptable" or even "attractive" to persons who do not have a disability.

The following are some general characteristics of medium- to high-tech user-friendly assistive device:
1. Provides multi-sensory cues and messages.
2. Operates as much as possible through gross, rather than fine, movements.
3. Is simple to operate and device complexity has been reduced.
4. Accommodates changes in the user.
5. Is as unobtrusive as possible.

Maggie's speech therapist, in discussing the design of communication devices, offers an example of the social aspects of device inconvenience:

> Socially and interpersonally, there can be difficulties. No piece of equipment on its own can bring social acceptance of the person. In fact, equipment can present its own social problems. For example, when a person uses a certain kind of typing device, the listener has to wait there for a very long time. Sometimes when they see the user approaching them, there's almost an avoidance reaction, "Oh, I don't want to get caught."

Levels of comfort with use, even around family members, vary widely. Feelings of being conspicuous leave many users feeling deviant and stigmatized. Rehabilitation engineers also acknowledge the inconvenience and potential stigmatizing effect of current devices:

> In some cases I've seen very good ideas developed, but they're so large and cumbersome that it takes hours for a person to set it up. Too, aesthetically [their size and shape, etc.] they may be so unusual that the person doesn't feel comfortable using them. People usually opt for the easy way out. If something has to be set up in a special way, if it's somewhat complex and it takes some time to do it, those are deterrents to use for all but the super-motivated. How would we like to be able to speak only after our device was set up? And we wouldn't want to have to wait to talk until our device was repaired.

A device that looks unusual and does not meet the user's real needs and desires is one that will end up stored in the closet.

Service delivery. Assistive technologies are not used if other supports for use are unavailable. For example, a communication device will go unused if the user is not provided training in how to use it. Persons in remote and rural areas may be unfamiliar with many devices because they haven't been exposed to them. Often persons with disabilities may not have access to peers or trained professionals to help them learn to use their new devices properly. If individuals have not received training in the limitations of hearing aids, for example, it is not uncommon for them to abandon them when they discover that perfect hearing is not restored. Similarly, users of communication devices need to learn the skills necessary for conversational and interactional use. Training cannot just focus on device operation. Often the technical aspects of rehabilitation have become so complex that specialists have de-emphasized the personal, emotional and social factors that facilitate technology adoption and use. The curriculum for training technologists leaves precious little room for courses in psychology, other social sciences, and the humanities.

While technical specialists may lack skills in human service delivery, rehabilitation professionals who do not perceive themselves as technically skilled may avoid learning about new technologies, downplay the usefulness of the devices, and fail to present them as viable options. If professionals have had unpleasant experiences matching consumers with technologies, or participated in too many overly technical workshops, they may have become soured on educational programs designed to increase, update, or broaden their own technical skills.

Users may be unwilling to request training or other assistance. As the quote from Brian indicated earlier in the section on "Personality and Temperament," a person with low self-esteem is not apt to be assertive about their needs. While many individuals remain uninformed about the options available to them, others are not accustomed to being assertive and for this reason may hesitate to ask for the assistance to which they are entitled. As one rehabilitation professional notes, training in device use is very important for both users and their family members and caretakers:

> The technology itself requires a lot of training [for] not only the user but the caregivers — because the caregivers have to learn how to problem-solve if there's a sudden malfunction of the equipment. We also need to start training those informal technicians, such as the neighborhood electrician, who are called upon to troubleshoot devices.

Equally important is the availability of a back-up system:

Technology brings more breakdowns and frustration as a result of that. Sometimes the downtime for repairs can be very long so a person needs access to a back-up system of some sort.

Maggie, who now uses a communication device but who used a manual communication board during our first meeting, has a speech therapist who made a similar point:

> Assistive device use should only be encouraged and recommended when the potential user can tolerate technology breakdown or downtime and utilize other compensatory skills and techniques. It also frequently occurs that a school will supply a communication system of some type for a student's use that has to be left there at the end of the day. Then the student has to go home and use a different means of communicating.

In addition, people develop and change. Unless they have ongoing access to rehabilitation professionals, they may stop using a device when all it may require to become useful again is some small adjustment or modification. Children, in particular, outgrow devices (either physically or developmentally) and need to be able to get upgrades or more developmentally appropriate devices. Another problem is the overgeneralization of devices. Therapists who have had success with a particular device with one or two clients — or who have close ties to certain vendors — may prescribe that device too frequently, believing it to have wider application than it in fact has.

Funding for devices. Funding for assistive technologies is problematic. Payors of assistive technology typically look at a 5-6 year product lifespan, which penalizes those active users who wear out their devices more quickly. Not only are limited funds available for devices, but agency policies often work at cross purposes so that many persons fall between the cracks. If a person is unemployed, does not qualify for vocational or educational assistance, cannot obtain private health insurance, and is not medically eligible for Medicaid or Medicare, there are few remaining options other than university-based programs with research funding and private philanthropy.

High-functioning individuals can be served at less expense than those with more severe disabilities who are low-functioning. Since funding, trained personnel, and equipment are limited, the general practice is to utilize the available pool of resources to help as many high-functioning persons as possible maintain or enhance their functioning, rather than exhaust already limited resources on relatively few low-functioning individuals. Persons not in the labor force may be unable to get the equipment they need in order to be employable. Another problem occurs when there is an overemphasis on assistive technologies in the workplace, because it sends a signal to persons with disabilities that they cannot expect to be employed unless they can do everything a non-disabled employee can do. It reinforces the attitude on the part of employers and fellow workers that people with disabilities present difficult problems requiring high-tech solutions. As noted in an issue of *Newsletter for Industry* (published by the President's Committee on the Employment of People with Disabilities), an airport guidance system — strips of wire under the carpeting in airports which give audio guidance signals to blind travelers equipped with a special receiver — lead people to believe that blind people can't adapt to the world around them without such accommodations. On the other hand, for an employer who believes mobility is a central problem for blind employees, such a system may serve to show that blind persons can be in jobs which require travel.

Cost-effectiveness. The cost-effectiveness of assistive technologies is a primary concern as we've entered the 21st century. If a low-cost device has only limited uses, or requires the same number of man-hours to use as the next cheapest alternative, or provides no gain in independence, then it's not cost-effective. A very expensive device, such as a reading machine for a person who is blind, may pay for itself in 2 to 5 years just in the amount of money saved in readers' fees. Beyond this, it allows for greater independence and flexibility than a human reader; its varied applications and capabilities make it a quite reasonable — even bargain — investment.

Another example of the kinds of trade-offs that figure into the calculations of cost-efficient and cost-effective approaches to rehabilitation is provided by Dudek, writing in 1985 and using costs at that time. For $500, a 30-year-old male who is a dual-leg amputee can have a manual wheelchair, which may result in a gain of 15% of the lower limit of "normal mobility." His personal care and transportation needs over a 30-year lifespan yield a total cost of about $420,500 (in 1985 figures). A power wheelchair with a cost of $15,000 could give him 30% of the lower limit of normal mobility, and he may then only need a part-time attendant, which would drop the 30-year lifespan costs to $375,000. If this individual is provided with prosthetic limbs and therapy, he may regain 75% of the lower limit of "normal mobility" at a cost of $45,000. He will have considerable autonomy, would require limited personal care, and could drive an adapted automobile — at a total cost over 30 years of $90,000.

In this case, rehabilitation (what Dudek considers the provision of prosthetic limbs) is preferable to maintenance (the provision of a manual or power wheelchair) because it minimizes costs. When there are several possible alternative paths to a specific goal, small investments in rehabilitation may be as effective as (and much more efficient than) large investments in maintenance. But this effectiveness requires use of recommended devices. What if this person doesn't use his prosthetic limbs? What if he only wants to use them part of the time (since such prostheses are often uncomfortable or even painful) and use a wheelchair the rest of the time?

The rehabilitation of many individuals may not be as cost-efficient as maintenance combined with environmental modifications. For example, equipping a hundred dual amputees with prosthetic limbs in a large metropolitan area may be less cost-efficient than providing them with wheelchairs and smoothly paved streets and buildings with ramps (which will also benefit people pushing carts and delivery persons with handtrucks). But when an environment cannot be easily or cost-efficiently modified, it may be less costly to rehabilitate and equip relatively few individuals.

Models of costs and benefits say a lot about comparisons among numbers, but little about *people*. While such models do have an important role, they should always be critically evaluated as to why they were done, by whom, how well, and for what purpose. Their value in providing a broad overview for budgeting and policymaking should rarely come at the expense of decisions regarding individuals' needs, preferences, and quality of life.

PRACTICAL STEPS TO ACHIEVING A GOOD MATCH OF PERSON AND TECHNOLOGY

While rehabilitation settings are very responsive to the physical needs of individuals with disabilities, there is frequently less attention given to the individual's emotional and social needs and preferences. Addressing the Milieu, Personality, and Technology factors helps identify desirable changes to foster device use and enhance the user's quality of life. This will reduce device abandonment and decrease premature or inappropriate device recommendations. Documenting a person's functioning before and after the device is used can (a) help provide the rationale for funding a device or training for that device, (b) demonstrate an individual's improvement in functioning over time, and (c) help organize information typifying the needs of an organization's consumers.

Some tough, but important, questions that should be asked every individual considering the purchase or adoption of any assistive technology are:
1. What do you — not someone else — think you need?

2. What is it exactly that makes you think that? What's led you to that decision or opinion?
3. What is a typical day like for you — from the time you get up to the time you go to bed at night? Describe your activities, the people you usually see, the places you go.
4. What do you wish a typical day will be like one year from now? Five years and ten years from now?
5. What do you see as being most useful and helpful to you now? In the future in achieving your goals?
   After identifying assistive technology usage from the above 5 questions, the next series of questions should ask:
6. What do you want to do?
7. Where? In what different environments or settings?
8. What assistance is already available in those settings? What will assistive device use add to — or take away from — that assistance?
9. What changes in lifestyle are involved? For whom?
10. What non-technical solutions are available? What are their pros and cons?
11. What's the lowest level technical solution that will meet your needs and achieve the goal?
12. How well will it function in the various situations where you will use it?

To assist consumers in determining the desirability of an AT for their use and then comparing their device options, a group of peer mentors working through the Regional Center for Independent Living (Rochester, NY) prepared a workbook containing guiding questions to consider. Portions of this workbook are included in Appendix B.

Targeting a Good Match: A Review and Organization of Key Influences on AT Use

Figure 8-2 is a graphic representation of a more complete and complex process which complements Figure 7-3. It is the foundation of the MPT assessment process, so let me explain it in more detail, going step by step, as it summarizes the discussion to this point.

The target in the center circle is the most appropriate match of user and assistive technology. As discussed, there are three major areas of influence on this match:

1. Characteristics and resources of the person.

2. Characteristics and requirements of the milieu or environments of use.

3. Characteristics of the technology itself.

While the characteristics and resources of the person will ultimately determine the consumer's choice of one product over a competing one, all of these influences interact with and determine one another. That is why the outermost circle reflects an on-going, iterative, dynamic process of user-product evaluation, selection, accommodation (or adjustment), and use.

Characteristics and Resources of the Person

The most important influence on the decision to use an AT is the nature of the functional need for this particular device. Given the user's physical capacities, does the product have the desired portability/transportability and can the person use it without undue fatigue or stress? These are examples of questions that need to be answered and which can vary according to the person's lifestyle and the degree to which one has the desire to use it and has adjusted to the need for AT use. Other key factors are the user's age and gender. We know that even very young children have clear preferences for devices that will not make them look different from their peers. This is also true for parents who may resist the idea of their child using an AT and will try to get by without it. Research with adolescent (non-disabled) girls conducted by Carol Gilligan (1992) shows that with the onset of adolescence, the girls stopped being assertive and confident and started becoming more reflective, tentative, and reluctant. For adolescent girls with disabilities, these characteristics may result in their being excluded from decisions regarding assistive technologies and other matters which affect their lives, thus perpetuating the belief that they are passive and technically incompetent. Brown (1996) provides a good summary of many of the issues facing adolescents with disabilities (e.g., self-image and independence) in her article on perceptions and use of functional electrical stimulation-augmented standing by adolescents with spinal cord injuries.

The July 1996 report of the National Council on Disability acknowledges that both younger and older women with disabilities face dual barriers and continue to be dually disenfranchised — first, from having a disability and second, from being poorly matched with a product they need to use regularly. This thesis has been discussed for more than a decade (e.g., Willmuth & Holcomb, 1993) with little change in the status of women with disabilities in today's society.

As they age, consumers have a clear preference for products that they do not have to think about (are easy to care for and maintain and which accommodate them, not vice versa). When presented with a choice, consumers will select assistive devices, as they do with any product, according to characteristics that satisfy their preferences. Therefore, as the diversity of both products and the users of those products expands, it is increasingly important to be able to understand the different needs and preferences among users and to provide each consumer with the products he or she needs and wants. That preferences vary is not only crucial for providers to understand when matching a person and a device, but also for manufacturers and vendors to consider as they design and market their products. In the case of many ATs, users may not have choice over whether or not to use it, but can exercise choice in their selection of style and the environments in which they use it.

Characteristics and Requirements of the Milieu (Environments of Use)

When we think about people with disabilities living and working in different environments, we are accustomed to thinking primarily in terms of the physical accessibility of those environments. But environments have other characteristics that are equally deserving of attention. For example, different environments tend to draw people of varying ages, cultural backgrounds, educational and leisure interests, and so on. The attitudes of the individuals in an environment towards the inclusion of persons with disabilities is good information to have in order to make inclusion as smooth as possible. Political and economic characteristics of environments is typically considered when comparing policies and services between different countries, but even different regions of the U.S. will have distinctions that affect available resources to persons with disabilities. Because the word *environment* is so often viewed in terms of only physical accessibility, I frequently use the French word *milieu* because it more adequately connotes the totality of physical/architectural and attitudinal differences characterizing the environments in which individuals live, work, and socialize.

Characteristics of the Technology

Many ATs come in different sizes, styles, and with options regarding features and accessories. Key considerations when selecting an AT include how well it performs and how comfortable the person feels in using it. In other words, it must do the job for which it is intended without putting the user at undue risks for conditions secondary to use. The proliferation of options in product functions, features, and accessories make it increasingly complex — and important — for consumers to be able to understand the differences among available choices and to have the information they need and want in order to make informed product selections.

People select assistive technologies based, first, on their agreement that the device is needed, then how well the general product category satisfies their functional needs and preferences, and finally according to a particular product's attractiveness and appeal. Over time, the continued use of an AT will be determined by its on-going performance and usefulness for the user in actual situations of use. If it continues to meet the individual's performance expectations and is easy and comfortable to use, then a good match of person and technology has been achieved. This will continue dynamically through a cycle of device and feature evaluation, selection, accommodation, and use in various environments.

SUMMARY

Key points associated with less than optimal technology use is a failure to consider the user's opinions and preferences in device selection — in other words, *the individual's needs, preferences and expectations were not adequately or thoroughly assessed.* When selecting a device for a person's use, it is important to keep in mind the three primary MPT domains:

Milieu

Personality (preferences, outlook, adjustment, attitude and mood)

Technology

Only during a thorough assessment can the best judgment be made regarding:

- Need for an AT (and equipping the person) versus modifying the environment or the family's responses and support

- Impact of related limitations (such as low vision for the user of an augmentative communication system)

- Balance of functional *capabilities* and *limitations*

- Level of need for training and the identification of settings for trial use (home, work, school)

• Most cost-efficient device for the user in terms of usability and aesthetics

• Extent to which the device is meeting the consumer's needs at follow up and the existence of any undesirable secondary effects

The ultimate outcome of the assistive technology service delivery process is enhanced functioning, self-concept, and quality of life. If the device doesn't do that, it will not be used. Nor, perhaps, should it.

CHAPTER NINE

Battles Fought and Won, Battles Waged and Lost

Fasten your seatbelts. It's going to be a bumpy night.
— Spoken by **BETTE DAVIS** in *All About Eve* (1950)

Each of the individuals whose experiences, ideas, frustrations, and hopes are shared in this book has continued to undergo change during the years since our first contact. Physically there have been ups and downs, not only for the individuals themselves, but also for their family members and caregivers. For many, their family composition and dynamics changed over time. In addition to new emotional stresses, time presented challenges socially as well as economically. There remain continuous battles to be fought — small and large.

BATTLES WON

Jim. In 1998, Jim still worked for the insurance company. For some time he reported that he had become "fed up," saying, "Behind closed doors, they say no one like me can get a promotion." Part of his job was ADA compliance, and he believed they were angry with him "for pushing the ADA issues — equipment, equal opportunities. If they keep within their budget, they get a bonus. ADA costs money. If I go away, all of ADA goes away there."

"They also say my speech is interfering with the job, but I have proof it's not an issue." In response to his request/demand for equal pay, they downgraded his job from accountant to clerk and he resented working with "people with just high school diplomas. They changed my group and now I am isolated." About his supervisor he said "He doesn't know anything." He lost his private office and had to share a room with two other people, feeling "pushed into a corner" by himself.

In 1996, Jim said to me, "They can't fire me, but they can make my life miserable. But I'm not totally whipped yet. My sister and I are talking about starting a business in Michigan. It's time for a change."

In the spring of 1999, Jim called and told me he had just been fired. He also shared with me the fact that he had just recently "got out of detox." Jim had become an alcoholic, which he attributed to stress at work and from his father's death. "In January, I tried to commit suicide, but I was reaching out. Later in January I went into detox and got into AA [Alcoholics Anonymous] and that was the best thing I ever did. There's nothing they won't do for me. I'm also in counseling." Jim, now 44, has yet to find a lasting relationship but says, "I have a very strong feeling that I will find the right person. I already have two possibilities in AA. And I have a friend, Liz, who is executive director of the local independent living center. At one point I wanted to marry her. She talks the talk, but doesn't walk the walk. She's too controlled by her parents."

When things did not work for Jim as he wished, he maintained his tendency to attribute this to others rather than to any behaviors or short-comings in himself. He remained critical of others with disabilities and yearns for a solid and lasting relationship, which has so far remained an unfulfilled dream.

When Jim and I talked in September 2004, he told me that has not had a drink in a long time and has given up driving. Because he is aging, he now has a personal assistant "for the first time in my life." He moved into a brand new condo that he designed himself and, with pride, described the cathedral ceiling in his living room and the layout of the kitchen. He is in the process of preparing for an open house on the occasion of his 50th birthday.

Jim has not had a job since he left the insurance company. As we talked it was obvious, however, that he was feeling in control of a life that he finds positive and satisfying. In fact, he said, "I'm more content now than I've ever been."

Brian. Brian, too, had yet to find the "right girl" in 1999. But to Brian, his life is complete as he leads an active, personally enjoyable lifestyle.

After he had moved to California, I was in San Francisco for a conference and called Brian to see if it was possible for us to get together. He lived about sixty miles from where I would be staying, but offered to drive to the nearest station and then "BART in" to meet me at my hotel.

I recognized him instantly from across the hotel lobby. He was leaning over reading a book and was wearing a tie-dyed shirt, pea jacket, necklace and jeans. His hair was even longer now, and he wore it tied back in a ponytail. He appeared as tall and lanky as ever.

The first thing he shared with me was a recent experience he had had standing up (he had been held in a vertical position by straps). I asked what it had been like, after ten years. "Like seeing the ocean for the first time, it was that great."

Then Brian announced his plan to go back to school to study computer animation in addition to ushering at a local theater, continuing to tutor students in math, and visiting schools to teach young people "about what people with disabilities are really like."

Shared Adventures started with Brian's sit-ski experiences in 1985. The help he needed to ski (described in Chapter One) and for getting into a kayak, in a sailboat, on a surfboard, etc. was a situation he knew he shared with others with disabilities. He brought Shared Adventures with him to Santa Cruz, and made it a non-profit organization in 1994. In 2004, it serves over 1,000 people a year in 41 different activities that can be on any day and any time of the day. For example, an art class on Monday mornings, or sailing Thursday afternoons. Activities include group kayaking, surfing, sailing, climbing, hiking, para-sailing, scuba diving, skydiving, bird watching, hiking in the redwoods, and bicycling trips for people of all abilities. In Brian's words:

> Shared Adventures enriches the lives of all participants. Each person assumes a role either as a student, assistant, instructor or coordinator. People with or without disabilities work together equally; it's not the case that those without disabilities help those with disabilities. Our goals are to promote personal growth and development, encourage social interaction among all participants, increase cooperation and decision-making skills, improve problem-solving and leadership skills, and help people acquire outdoor skills and environmental awareness. We focus on capabilities, not "disabilities," and seek people who are optimistic and willing to take risks. Participants include those who are non-disabled, who have hearing or vision loss, mobility impairments, and learning and developmental disabilities.
>
> The list of activities will continue as time goes on. So, as you can see, my life can get a little busy.

Brian has an attitude, a philosophy, that life is meant to be lived to the fullest and that one should take both the positives and negatives in stride and keep moving onward. For Brian, this philosophy has been his lifeline and it has not wavered since he and I first met. While very close to his family and friends, he is not dependent on them for day-to-day support. He uses a combination of personal assistance and ATs.

> I still only need personal assistance for getting in and out of bed and doing chores around the house. I hire a few good people to come in at certain times of the day to help. With this, I'm able to get the best quality care I need.

Brian has figured out the blend of services he needs to conserve energy, but also achieve independence. In comparing his independence before his injury to now, he says, "My two legs and two motorcycle wheels have turned into a four-wheel motorized chair. That chair is now my freedom and independence. And, here I am, living life to its fullest."

Since moving to California, Brian has pursued his recreational interests "with a vengeance." He has a certificate in sailing and one in scuba diving. He has tried para-sailing, surfing, and white-water rafting. He continues his interest in sit-skiing and kayaking. He had a bungee-jumping experience from a hot air balloon which he particularly enjoyed:

Two tether ropes were hooked to the basket so it would reach one height and stop. Three people could fit at one time. The first jumper got in and the balloon went up to 150 feet. The jumper squatted on the rim of the basket and leapt off as if he were doing a swan dive into a pool. He did a freefall until he got to the end of the bungee cord, which caused him to stop 100 feet later, and then up he went again 50 feet, and so on like something on a rubber band. A few minutes later he came to a stop and the pilot lowered the balloon to where a team of people were there to catch him.

Forty people jumped that day, and not one chickened out. I heard them say, "It was the scariest thing I've ever done" and "It was the closest thing to death I've ever felt — you've got to do it." Well, after hearing that, I had to do it. I wore a harness around my shoulders and hips and my legs were strapped together. The director of the trip held me in a honeymoon carry. Then we went up to 150 feet and, before I had time to think what I was really doing up there, we left the balloon.

It's hard to describe that feeling of falling. I'm glad I did it but I don't think I'll do it again. Still, after that experience I feel like I can do anything.

You know, after my accident I kept a journal of events that evolved each day, positive or negative. Reading them now, the growth I see is mind-boggling. I owe my parents so much thanks. They played a big part in getting my feet back on the ground — so to speak!

I do look forward to a married life at some point. I still haven't found the right girl, but I have had several close girlfriend relationships. It takes time and understanding and, most of all, communication. My heart seems to speak first, and then my head follows. I don't know if that's good because there's always some hidden expectation and somebody ends up getting hurt. But without love in a dream, it'll never come true.

A few months passed, and then I received a letter from Brian. He started out talking about the Berkeley and Oakland fires and then, almost as a postscript, he wrote,

Oh yeah, I ended up in the hospital for five days with pneumonia and a collapsed lung. The flu hit hard here and I was a victim. No sleep for three days and my lungs felt like they were filled with a gallon of fluid. In comparison, it feels like the wind getting knocked out of you. It brought back a lot of old memories and made me realize again how lucky I am to be alive. Perhaps this will become a new chapter, or my third life. Who knows ... what a strange trip it's been.

For the past week it's been sunny and 75 degrees. My new parrot and I just got back from a walk to the beach. She's getting to be a real ham on our trips. She has a funny whistle and loves to be held by the people that stop and talk with us — especially the ones with earrings.

A few months later, Brian's stamina and resilience were put to the test again. While he was driving on Highway 1, his parrot was having some difficulty which caused Brian to glance at and reach toward her. He "lost control of the van and went into a bridge. I broke my leg, three ribs, and I have a punctured lung."

His resilience was tested yet again in 1998 — several times. Brian uses e-mail to stay in touch, and what follows are excerpts from e-mail letters he sent over a period of approximately one year. While, like everyone, he has experienced ups and downs, his pendulum swings reach both lower and higher than most people's do.

[1.] Life is treating me well. At times there are things that come up and it feels like someone is testing my patience. I get stuck in a situation and I have to figure out how I'm going to get out of it. One example was getting stuck in the back alley of where I work. It was a Saturday and raining when the lift on my van stopped 3 inches above the ground. I tried to get off and the whole lift went up because of the weight of the van. The rain was coming down hard and I was there at least 20 minutes before a car came in the alley. My shoulders were touching my knees as my chair was almost at a 45 degree angle to the ground. They asked if I needed any help! Um ... ! They helped me get in a sitting position and I was fine after that. I was a little emotionally shook up, though.

I'm blessed with a lot of beautiful women in my life. Not being committed to any one of them except I allow them my kind heart and if they don't see that then I guess they don't belong with me. I'm satisfied with that. Getting involved in a single committed relationship has been too painful. So I have many great ones.

[2.] I have a new job! It's for a residential facility for young people with disabilities. My first day was Wednesday. The Admission Intake person took me on a tour and talked to me about the building, residents, staff, therapists, doctors, etc. That was about 45 minutes. I then hung out for another hour and a half talking with the residents and getting a feel for what it would be like if I had to live there. A lot of stuff going on. I wish I could show you the activities schedule. From 10:00 am to 6:30 pm seven days a week there's always something going on.

There are over seventy young people and most all of them have pretty good thinkin' brains. I was talking to this guy Bill who collapsed in a field and is now paralyzed from the waist down. No one knows why. He needed so much to talk to me. That's one thing they don't have are counselors. They have Ph.D. shrinks to figure out meds but nothing like what I can offer. Which is information on how I got to where I am.

This is a perfect job for me. My own hours at $20/hr. But I have to play my cards right. I don't want to lose my benefits.

[3.] On Friday, the owners of where I live said it's time for me to start looking for a new place. When she said it my heart hit the floor. At first I was in disbelief but in a way not surprised. They have to do major repairs on the roof in the front house (I live in the back) which has been leaking in their bedroom all winter. They can't live in the house while the roof is being repaired. Plus I know they're eyeing this place for her Mom who is living in Virginia. It's a perfect guesthouse when relatives come into town. And they have a lot. So it's going to be great for them.

Not so great for me. But in a way I need to expand too.

I really haven't given it much thought about what I'm going to be looking for yet. I've been in this place almost eight years. A lot of stories shared in this house. Some great times and not so great. I'm sad but this is a start of a new beginning. I wonder where my new home will be? Wish me some good luck.

[4.] I moved in with two friends Saturday. Nice place. Two dogs, garden, firepit. I feel very welcome here. It's good size room and closet space. So far I have my bed, computer desk, office desk, small file cabinet and a bunch of other stuff.

Been having some heartbreaking experiences. A small one bedroom accessible cottage fell through. It could have worked but I didn't get it. It was a real nice place, too. Every other place I have called or checked out has been inaccessible. A lot of people are looking for a place to live too. So, I have a lot of competition. On top of not finding a place, Cindy and I are no longer together. A double whammy. I'm very heartbroken but life goes on. She was my best friend and we had some great times together. I feel grateful we were together. I'm sure we'll be keeping in touch. I have to remind myself it takes time to heal.

[5.] I've got my own place!

The site manager called yesterday and said I can start moving in two months from now. What a load off my mind. On the 8th I go in and fill out a bunch of paperwork.

The place is a one bedroom, living room, dining room, kitchen, with sliding glass doors, small yard and garden. I only have to pay a 1/3 of my income. Four months of looking...

Thanks for keeping your fingers crossed. I bought a new full size bed, futon couch and microwave. The old bed must be over twelve years old because I bought it used ten years ago. My paintings and silk screens are getting put up on the walls. It's really a beautiful place. My new home. Wish you could come visit.

[6.] I was hanging out Saturday night just taking it easy and around 10:00 PM I emptied my leg bag. My urine was red. I had a couple of antibiotics left over from the last time I had one. I took those and drank a lot of water. 11:00 PM Alan came over to help me into bed. At that time I was sweating and felt a little feverish. I got horizontal and my head started pounding. I started shaking and was not feeling well at all. This happened to me last year and my old housemate (studying to be a paramedic) helped me to the Emergency Room. The doctor said if that happens again, don't wait, have someone bring you in or call 911. Well, this time I called 911. A fire truck and ambulance came. I was having a hard time even speaking. Pretty scary. In the ER they did all the things they do. By the time the doctor came about an hour and a half later I stopped shaking. The nurse came in with a pain killer shot but I said no way. I was starting to feel better anyway. They let me rest. About an hour later the nurse came in and said how are we going to get you home. Alan wasn't feeling good when he came over that night so I said the ambulance. They got me into bed at 4:30 AM and I slept until noon. Been resting and drinking water all day. Feeling a lot better. Being healthy is so important and I am. It's weird how something like that can sneak up on me.

[7.] It was a bladder infection. I'm on an antibiotic now and see the doctor tomorrow. Still weak and have a little fever. Drinking a lot of H2O and taking it easy. Thanks for writing. Feels nice to have such great support and I'm happy to be alive...

[8.] I found out I was picked for the 61st Annual Junior Chamber of Commerce TOYA Award. TOYA stands for Ten Outstanding Young Americans. I get flown with a guest, all expenses paid, to Washington, DC in January. I will receive a trophy and a medallion.

They're going to put together a video of pictures, newspaper clippings and other video coverage to have as an introduction before I go on stage. Over 800 people are supposed to be attending. It's a full agenda that starts Friday night, all day Saturday into the night and Sunday morning. You would not believe the people who have been selected over the past 60 years. Clinton ('79), Gore (80'), JFK ('46), Ralph Nader ('66) Christopher Reeve ('81). I got fitted for a tuxedo today. I'm still pinching myself to see whether or not this is just a dream.

But let me get over my bladder infection first! Been having migraine headaches when I pee sometimes. Having a blood test done tomorrow and more extensive test with a urologist on Monday.

Life is such a trip.

Part of "living life to the fullest" for Brian is being able to take as many risks as a person without a disability. While the consequences of his pneumonia and bladder infections gave him complications a non-disabled person would not have, he much prefers to exercise choice and to take these risks.

Brian has had his spinal cord injury for more than half his life. Over that time, he has maintained a consistent belief in the value of thinking positively and living life to the fullest. In 2002, he had another serious case of pneumonia and ended up in the hospital. But he won that battle, as well as many others during the past few years. Based on all that he has experienced and learned, I asked Brian what advice he would give to someone with a new spinal cord injury.

Get as much support as possible in the community, the department of rehab, go to school, keep your brain from dwelling on what you don't have and do the things you can do for yourself. Strive to be as independent as you can be — and get outdoors and explore. Try to get into a group setting, as least some of the time. I know a lot of people are introverted. I like my alone time, too. So find that balance of time with others and time alone. Get creative and find some hobbies to keep your mind busy. Keep your body in shape and work out. I've tried so hard over the years. I use my pedal-in-place every morning to keep my legs moving and I've used it everyday since I got it nine years ago. I also go to a community college to work out with weights, stand up, participate in dance, and adaptive swimming.

Eating well is important... eat your vegetables. I don't mean to sound like a mom, but you'll feel better about yourself if you don't overindulge in liquor and you eat well and exercise. And you'll have more energy. I usually do a good balancing act in taking care of myself. But I'm also a good example of what happens when I don't follow that advice, which I can tend to do from time to time. This weekend I outdid myself. I stayed out late, I got up early, I went to church and then I met with friends and went to a meeting and out to dinner, drank a margarita and it all added up. So when Monday came around I had a bladder infection.

I think a big thing is try to fix what's not working for you. If you're not happy with something, then try to do something about it. Get into a support group or two. Explore what's on the Internet and books. What's helped me, too, if I'm feeling down and in a rut and I need some extra help, I'll go to family services and see a counselor and talk with them about who I am and what I'm doing. That works for me. It's really important to not give up.

As Brian had said to me years before, "I'll keep trying until I find a way that works." It is certainly the case that Brian has to think about living with a spinal cord injury and achieving his dreams in new and different ways, but he never made his injury his major focus. He does what he can for himself, but other than that he really doesn't care what's out there. For example, Brian told me that he volunteers his time to Shared Adventures in exchange for his expenses being paid.

> I can't claim any money because if I do that then they cut me off, the system. I can't work because my benefits will go down, my housing will go up, and my medical will disappear.

When I asked for his opinion of the Ticket to Work[1] program, he said,

> I've heard about it, but I really don't know about it. I'm not sure what that's all about.

That statement was an indication to me that he is not fully aware of, nor involved in, the system today. What is clear is that he sees the years ahead as intriguing and exciting, and not something to feel anxious about or to fear.

Chris. Now a retired vocational rehabilitation counselor, Chris continues to thoroughly enjoy her retirement; she says that "getting older adds aches here and there but is far better than the alternative." When I told her how much she continues to be missed and that no one has been able to satisfactorily fill her shoes, she says, "There have been two after me — but times and rules change, so no comparison is fair."

Maggie. Like Brian, Maggie has been able to bounce back from a serious health incident. In 1994 she was ready to try employment again, even though she did not believe her prospects were very good. In her 1994 Christmas letter, she gave this update:

> Just want you to know Theresa and I are thinking of you. She is writing this short note for me as I am busy submitting an application for employment in a strange, but interesting city. I will not get the job, nor will we move. It is a great dream, though, and if it does come true, you will know next year. Nothing much happened this year. Mother is doing exceptionally well, I think, though she is in pain. Now, at least, she can get out and has maintained most of her activities.

Maggie and Theresa serve on the boards of a number of disability organizations, are active churchgoers, and are advocates for disability rights. In 1998, they moved into their own "brand new" house. It is fully accessible and features an open floor plan to make it easier for Maggie to get around. Theresa is particularly pleased that she can now have a garden.

Since 1986 when Maggie was learning Prentke-Romich's *Express* communication system (described in Chapter Two), she has gone to the *Light Talker* to the *Liberator* and in 2003, to the *Pathfinder*. Maggie laughingly calls herself a "poster child for AAC."

In the summer of 2003 Maggie and Theresa drove from their home to Pittsburgh for a conference on the Pathfinder. They called to say that from Pittsburgh they wanted to drive up to see me. They arrived as scheduled and I met them at their motel.

Right away we had to call technical support at Prentke-Romich because Maggie's *Pathfinder* was being repaired and she had a loaned replacement. Theresa and I were given trouble-shooting support over the phone in clear step-by-step instructions. Theresa was very proficient, but it required trials with different strategies to get it going again. We had to check the battery, turn it on and off, etc. But throughout their visit, Maggie rarely used it. Even though using a manual board is no longer an option for her due to paralysis after her neck surgery, she preferred to have Theresa speak for her, saying, "It's just easier that way." She told me she only uses her *Pathfinder* for presentations and for communicating with strangers.

Maggie paid the $8,000 cost for her *Pathfinder* with her own funds.

> To have Medicare pay for it, I would have had to wait for the *Liberator* to wear out and confirmed to be non-repairable, and I didn't want to wait.

Her neck surgery resulted in Maggie's right and left arms becoming paralyzed ("actually, my entire upper torso is paralyzed, and I had trouble breathing for a while"). She has had botox injections to relax the muscles so that her arms and hands don't lock in around her face. After her neck surgery, Maggie got very depressed and said she would have killed herself but she didn't want to leave Theresa alone.

Theresa drove us around flawlessly in their 6-year old Ford van, which now has about 124,000 miles on it. Maggie uses a lift out the back of the van that Theresa operates.

Maggie has an Invacare Torque SP power wheelchair that fully reclines. She sits up quite high in it because of the size of the battery under it. She likes to move fast, but has sporadic control of the chair. She kept running into things (planters, wastebaskets, knocked the filter off their motel heating unit) partly because she can't see them as she sits so high with her feet extended out, and partly because she has an aggressive reaction to obstacles in her path. Theresa repeatedly yells at her (somewhat sternly), "Maggie, be careful." But when Maggie does run into something, Theresa just laughs. This is characteristic of Theresa's temperament: Nothing really bothers her, or for long.

Maggie is now 60 years old and Theresa is 52. Maggie wore sandals and stockings, white slacks, and a striped white and pink top and white and pink earrings. Her thinning hair has been colored a light red and it was flattened in the back because of her head pressing against the neck rest on her wheelchair. She is very thin and ate little when we went out for lunch, which she attributes to some extent to her teeth: "They were ruined from using a mouth stick." Her fillings are falling out and she says they can't be re-done. "I want implants." Theresa, too, has problems with her teeth as a result of TMJ [TemporoMandibular Joint syndrome which is associated with pain on opening or closing your mouth, eating and chewing food, and even speaking] and she also has carpal tunnel syndrome. She had surgery on one hand; the other will be done soon. She is stocky, and wore an attractive short sleeve top and shorts.

Theresa has hearing loss in both ears and wears two hearing aids, but one is not working and she took out the other one because it hurt her ear. Theresa is capable and mature but then gets as excited as a child about going to see something new and different.

Theresa is very grateful to Maggie for the lifestyle she can now lead. Maggie is grateful for Theresa's help, loyalty and caring. For both, their relationship has resulted in a high quality of life neither would have achieved on her own.

Ann and Linda. Inadequate personal assistance created a crisis. In late May 1994, Linda fell four times while trying to get herself to the bathroom. She required back surgery as a result. When stabilized, Linda went to the hospital rehabilitation unit, but then her worst fears came true: She had to go into a nursing home for three months.

> I couldn't stay in rehabilitation. The nursing home was horrible. They didn't know what they were doing. But it was close to home and I managed to go home twice. Then, to make matters worse, Ann had a breast removed in August. She had cancer. I was in the nursing home at the time.
>
> Now we cannot get out very much. Both of us don't feel so good. Most of the time I'm frustrated. I can't help it. We don't have the help we need. We both are supposed to go to rehabilitation some days, but our aides don't show up on time to get us ready on time, so often we're late for rehabilitation.

In 2004, Ann and Linda are still living in their apartment, and doing well. A series of letters show how they, too, have satisfying lives in spite of a number of frustrations. A major part of their success is due to attitude – and fortitude. The following was written in January 2001 by Ann on her computer.

> We started a letter to you way before Christmas. One thing led to another. And that letter kind of went by the wayside. Now that I have a break from my volunteer job, I thought it a good time to get caught up on some letter writing. And I know you've been wanting to hear from us.
>
> Let me start by saying I had my name in for over a year to a foundation that distributes computers to disabled people who can't afford them. All of a sudden a few days after Christmas, I got a phone call that they had a computer for me. Not only that, but when I asked the girl who called me how I would get it, she said, "Well, actually I live three houses down from you." That was a big plus.
>
> A few days later she brought the computer over, set it up, and spent some time showing me how to use it. She said she'd give me a week to get used to it and then come back to see how I was doing. In the meantime, a friend came over who helped me even more. He had me doing very well but, for some reason, the computer wouldn't boot up after that. It so happened the girl from the foundation came back later that day, but she had no idea what happened. So a few days later she brought me another one.
>
> I am still having a hard time learning to use the computer. I took an 8-week computer class at the rehabilitation center, but I was very slow and didn't accomplish half of what I would have liked to. And I have a very hard time remembering. Unless everything is written down for me, I'm lost. Everyone tells me not to get frustrated. However, right now I am. It is really because I'm so far behind on everything. And losing a lot of stuff doesn't help, either.

The letter stops. Further down the page Ann typed *February 2001* and continued with the following:

> I want to explain what is going on with my computer. I'm still having a rough time operating it. What I'm thinking about now is trading my new one for the one I work on at my volunteer job. I'm not at all sure people will agree with my decision. But I feel this might be the best thing for me.
>
> If I remember right, you also asked about our help. Right now we have six people coming in at different times. And we are grateful for all of them. We wouldn't be here without their help. We celebrated our 19th year in our apartment this summer so, needless to say, we're very proud of ourselves.

In their Christmas 2002 letter, they wrote a lot about various family members and friends, but also shared the following experiences:

We are both pretty well, except for a lot of arthritis, which makes it harder to do things. Linda is still taking art classes at home and is now working on her third picture. This summer she saw the exhibit on Van Gogh and Gaugin. And we went to the theatre. The day we went it was raining, so we took a cab home. The wheelchair cabs are very nice, but they can only take one chair at a time.

One morning towards the end of July we were sitting out in the yard waiting for a ride when some lady grabbed Linda's purse and ran. Wow, talk about scared. All of her I.D.'s were gone. And it is a pain in the neck to get others. As this letter is being typed, she still hasn't got everything back.

The next Christmas letter from Ann and Linda (December 2003) was decidedly more upbeat in spite of the need to wait for new wheelchairs and the disappointment that comes with not having one's creativity rewarded as quickly as desired.

A very Merry Christmas and Happy New Year. Where in the world did the year go?

We still have six wonderful helpers who work very well together. When one can't come in, she'll call the other one. They all have their own way of doing things, and it gets very frustrating at times. But we love them all.

We are both waiting for new power chairs that recline. We were both fitted. However, Medicare is so slow, it might be a year before we get them. We'll let you know how it works out.

Linda is still enjoying her artwork and doing very well. I'm enjoying my writing, although not getting very far with it. I wrote one article for a book, and if it was accepted they'd pay me $100. However, I never heard anymore about it. I've also sent in some articles to Reader's Digest, but they haven't responded. So it's very difficult to make any money on writing.

That's about all the news for this year. We wish you the best for the coming year.

With advances in technology have come advancing years for the individuals in this book. Functional declines have occurred for many due to aging and recurrent health problems. Maggie now has more sophisticated devices as a result. And what worked for Linda and Ann ten, or even five, years ago cannot be expected to work now. Until they got the assistance they needed, Linda and Ann could not maximize their capabilities and achieve a satisfactory quality of life.

Brian, too, has had to obtain new assistive technologies due to changing needs. As he explained to me,

My body has been getting older and… I just turned 43… I don't have the energy level like before. I use a motorized chair, a van, computer, phone, all are technology at its finest. In 30 years my feet have gotten a little worse in terms of circulation. So I have a high-tech chair where my feet go over my head. It's sort of like a lazy-boy chair. I have a button on the right side of the chair and when I push it one way my legs elevate and when I push the button the other way, the chair tips back. With my feet up and reclining, I'm in a horizontal position. [Much like Maggie can do in her current wheelchair]. When I can recline the chair back and put my feet up and then chill out for a little bit, it's good for my body. But the chair hasn't been working right… the wires have been shorting out… and I'm a little frustrated.

Brian does have another wheelchair he can use and has always believed that, "It's important to have a back-up whenever possible." He also has a back-up van, both of which are "pretty old now."

BATTLES LOST

Chuck. For Chuck, life in 1999 had remained about the same. He had a temporary respiratory problem that required him to use oxygen, but said the last time he was in the hospital was two years ago.

I still get decubitus, but I heal at home. So far, so good. The last time I was there, managed care wanted to send me home but I talked them into keeping me longer.

It's getting worse and worse to get my normal supplies. It used to be that I could pick up the phone, get a prescription, and have my stuff sent to me. Now, with all the paperwork and everything, when I need something, it's such a hassle to try and get it. And I'm stuck with what's on the list for me. Any change would require a new prescription which might take a while to get.

He got out a little more, but said that the Americans with Disabilities Act had not resulted in many changes for him.

Not in my town. There are doorways you can't get in, much less worry about ramps. But, this is a small, rural town. Some stores have put up some plywood ramps, but not that much has been done. When I go to K-Mart or Wal-Mart, it's okay. Most of the time, when we go out to eat, it's to a fast food place, a high-volume place, and they're okay. Here in town, there are two restaurants. And one is accessible… sort of. I have to go in another door, where they bring in supplies and stuff, but… [M]y biggest problem still is where I live. Last year I went 6-7 months without a vehicle I could rely on. Little local trips were okay, but anything further, forget it. If I lived in the city, things would be better.

Chuck really would have liked something to do to "keep the grey matter going — like mentoring, research, whatever." He said he didn't want money, just expenses (like travel) covered.

In 2003 I received the news that Chuck's family situation had changed (he lived with his sister and brother-in law) and that he was now living in a skilled nursing facility. When I called to talk with him, I was told that he had just been taken to the hospital for pneumonia and was "trached." He died shortly after.

Butch. In 1991, Butch was getting out more and had built a new power wheelchair for himself.

> It took me three months to design the wheelchair the way I wanted it, to figure it all out. Everything is worked on such close tolerances, it's unbelievable. I did it my way, not somebody else's way. I know what I want to satisfy *me*. And if it satisfies me, then I'm all set. As of right now, I could have sold thirteen of them — right out from underneath me. One guy in the hospital wanted to buy it right on the spot. But I can't sell them... unless I can make a million dollars, I can't make a penny as I'm wrapped up in this Medicaid situation. I'm up against a rock and a hard place.

Having met with success in building his wheelchair, Butch then decided to try and customize his own vehicle — a truck that is the center of attention wherever it goes.

> It's the ultimate handicapped rig. This thing, I've put my life into designing it, and I did a lot of the work on it myself. I'm out all the time with it. Anyplace I want to go. I love going to Niagara Falls. I jump in my truck and go when I want. You know how in everyone else's van you go in and out the side door? In this truck I go right out the back, drive right in, pull right up to the steering wheel and drive away. Takes me all of 10 seconds and I'm gone. I put a passenger seat in it that's the most comfortable seat you could ever ride in. I sat here and I thought and thought and did everything I could possibly think of to do to it before I ever got it on the road. And now that it's on the road, it.... [Butch suddenly changed his train of thought.] It's painted pink and purple. Pink and purple stripes with a big purple heart in the center of the back door... it's the love truck. And you know what my license plate reads? "A GIMP." Around that I have a neon light behind it that lights it up purple. And at night it lights the whole back of the truck up bright purple. Oh, it's a hoot to see it.

Ironically, after all his gains, Butch found himself in the role of caregiver in 1995. His father became ill and this put a strain on the entire family, as Butch described:

> The pacemaker isn't doin' what they thought it would do for him. It got his heart stabilized, but he's gettin' old — he's 78 now. He's been through so much... the pacemaker can't take away all the troubles he's had. Now his heart'll be beatin' forever, but he's going to end up being a vegetable anyway because his mind is going. It's Alzheimer's. He'll be talking about one thing and then he's talkin' about something from 60 years ago and then he's back talkin' about something else and he never finishes up. Ma and I have to watch him 24 hours a day. Now he'll get up and walk out the door and he don't even know he's out the door. Ma can't control him. She tells him to do somethin', he ignores her. I tell him to do somethin', he'll do what I tell him. We're just sittin' here stuck. I ain't been able to get out of the house to go for a ride or nothin'. It's bad enough being in this shape, now I'm trapped. There's nothin' else we can do. We can't put Pop in a nursing home or we'll lose the house. And we can't afford paid help.

Butch's father died in 1996. Then his brother lost his job, and house as a result, and moved back in with Butch and his mother (who was now 75 years old, frail and had difficulty walking). Butch had gray hair in his long beard now, and developed an ulcer in his foot. "Now I'm just sittin' again. I've put on more than 100 pounds. I'll tell ya', this whole place [home] is so hard. I just stay up here in this room and watch TV. Hopefully, when this sore heals, I can get out again."

He said he was "stuck" again and seemed frustrated and angry at this turn of events. Acknowledging "turns in luck" had become his coping strategy.

> But that's life. You gotta play the hand you're dealt. This is our hand. That's what makes it life. It's a game. You never know what's going to happen next or what hand the other guy has. There are some destined to be lucky, others not.

Life remained much the same for Butch until a few years ago in March he had an overwhelming infection, his temperature was high, blood pressure was low, and he was semi-conscious. A visiting nurse and a physician went in to talk with him. Butch had four wounds on his legs and one on his buttock and said he wanted to die at home. With his mother and brother present, he said he did not want hospital care, and that he had a DNR order and a living will. He debrided his wounds with a pocket knife and often refused to have his temperature checked saying, "Why bother?" According to the visiting nurse, "He knew what was happening and it was one area he had control over." The psychiatric nurse went out to confirm that Butch's mother and brother were okay with it. Butch died 3 days later.

The family was in poverty and his mother went into a nursing home but "died because she didn't eat enough to stay alive." His brother now lives alone in the house with his two sons. He has diabetes which is "very brittle" (meaning his blood sugar is up and down and not in good control). On December 26, 2000 he had a motorcycle accident. According to the perspective of the visiting nurse, "Everyone in that family had a death wish."

Ken. Ken, a social worker with a spinal cord injury, was born and raised in the country. When we reconnected in 1995, he had been on a waiting list for an accessible apartment back in his hometown for over a year and was becoming frustrated.

> I want to go back to a rural area because I'm from a rural area and I can't get used to the city. Granted you have more accessibility to shopping and services, but I don't have family up here either. Since I do drive, I will have access to the city.
>
> In the beginning, I wouldn't have gone back to the country because it would have been more like giving up. But now I've gotten to the point where I think I don't have to prove anything to me or anyone else. So, to go back to the country isn't so much giving up as living in the atmosphere I want to live in.

Walking into Ken's apartment building in the city in March 1995, I was struck by how depressing it looked, compared to when I had first started meeting with him nine years previously. There were people loitering around the entrance and the wind had piled litter where once there were flowers and shrubs. A well-furnished, large, homey lounge area, designed for relaxed resident gatherings, had become an institutional group dining room. Nine years ago the largest population in residence were senior citizens; now I could not pick out any single, predominant group.

> Another reason I want to move is that, when I first moved in here, the atmosphere was more friendly. It has gone down because of drugs. And there is more crime. Just last week they busted a woman down the hall and her friends. There's a lot of cocaine use in the building. The — quote — "mentally ill" in this building I think are more recovering drug addicts,

and that's their disability. And they get in here because of that, but they're not recovering, they're still active. Plus, this is just a bad area of the city for drugs and crime.

Drugs and crime were just two of Ken's complaints about his neighborhood. He was very much concerned about his overall quality of life and that of the individuals he knows who have psychiatric and emotional disabilities. He related to me an incident he found particularly disturbing:

This building is funded by HUD, so everyone here has a disability or is married to a person with a disability. When you say "disabilities," it has to cover the full spectrum. We have elderly people and people with AIDS, mental illness, CP, spinal cord injuries, all living together.

It's not right to dump people in the community without backup services. It's very bad for them. We even had one person who died right here down in the lobby, and I think a lot of it was bad, or total lack of support. He had been here for many years, but he never had a lot of backup support for his mental illness. He was schizophrenic and also diabetic. And he sat down in the lobby and just died one night, apparently from a diabetic coma in his sleep. It was like something out of a movie. My neighbor, Bob, also a quad, and I share the same aide. He came in about 2:00 one morning and the nurse's aide was waiting for him and came in with him. They came in, and there's Tommy apparently sleeping. Sitting like he always does with his legs crossed and his head leaning back. But he never slept down there at night, only during the day. Now Tommy and Bob, these two guys had always harassed one another, so Bob goes over — now he'd had a couple of drinks — and says, "C'mon, Tommy, time to go to bed. Get up, get up." And he's shaking him. Tommy's not moving. The aide is there holding the elevator saying, "Let's go, Bob, leave Tommy alone. You need your sleep." Bob has Tommy's arm and he's waving it around saying, "Wave good-bye, Tommy."

Well, Tommy at that point had been dead for about three hours. But Bob couldn't feel that he was cold. Finally, Bob said something like, "Hey, Tommy, you dead or what?" And the aide got to thinking, 'Bob *has* been shaking him awful hard....' She went over and Tommy was dead. The security guard hadn't been around... he was up with one of the drug prostitutes. Needless to say, he lost his job. We all felt just terrible about Tommy. What they did to him was inhumane. And this is just an example of what happens when there is poor supervision. And with the government cutbacks, it's just going to get worse.

After our meeting in March, I didn't talk with Ken for several months. Then, in August, I received bad news. Ken was in the hospital again and was very ill. This hit me hard. Since Ken is a social worker, he speaks from the perspective of a consumer and a professional, and he has given me many insights over the years. The 22 years since his spinal cord injury gave him plenty of time to adjust to his injury and to reflect upon that adjustment, as he related in Chapter Seven.

This time, Ken's hospitalization was not due to respiratory problems or to a pressure sore (occurrences for which he had been hospitalized many times). This time it was for a new and very serious illness.

I visited him in the hospital and learned that after his pressure sore had healed, a check-up showed he had urinary and kidney problems. In fact, one kidney was not functioning. Exploratory surgery revealed a mass that turned out to be cancer. Then in mid-July, he had surgery to remove a kidney and his bladder. He was not given chemotherapy or radiation treatment because he was considered to be at too high a risk. (In addition to his spinal cord injury, Ken has 30% lung capacity.) After the surgery, Ken went back to his apartment in the city.

Then things deteriorated rapidly. Visiting him, I was told Ken had a 102-degree temperature. They also told me that because of his injury, Ken could not feel pain. The entire time I was there he was in and out of consciousness.

Ken was very thin and pale. He spoke in such a low, weak voice that I couldn't really hear or understand him. He kept saying, as if to reassure me, "I'm getting better." I didn't think he'd last a week.

The day after I saw him, Ken rallied. But that proved to be temporary. Ken died a week later in the hospital which is located less than one mile from his city apartment. Ken finally made it back to his hometown, but it was for his burial.

During Ken's eulogy, a minister said that Ken "is finally rid of that *body* of his — the one that gave him so many challenges." The people attending his service, over 100, heard that Ken was a quiet, contemplative person and very kind. Ken did not focus on *doing* as much as on *being*, and he was paid tribute as a good rehabilitation counselor, even though he never did get the actual degree.

When Ken was first injured, he would pull the sheet up over his head to hide from the reality of his injury and functional limitations. Then he went though periods of depression and substance abuse, as he described in Chapter Seven. The eulogist said that this was when Ken was "entombed." It took a while, but he brought himself into a "second life" of quiet strength and helpfulness to others.

Ken was injured at age 18 from a fall into ravine behind his house. At the time of death, he was 40 years old and 22 years post-injury. He is buried with his parents; I was told by his brother that the grave marker had been all made up for him years ago.

The October 11, 2004 issue of USA Today reported the death of Christopher Reeve, who received a high level spinal cord injury in 1995 and was battling a systemic infection due to a decubitus ulcer, and, ironically, another article on the initial results of a brain implanted device that can help persons with paralysis to independently run a computer with their "thoughts," The intrigue of neuron-based devices notwithstanding, Ken had issued a plea in Chapter Six for more attention to the "basic things." While much progress has been made in assistive technology devices and services, additional progress needs to be made in prevention and treatment programs for pressure sores, urinary tract and pulmonary infections.

As individuals with disabilities age, adjustments are required in their healthcare and assistive technologies. With the managed health care system's current emphasis on cost containment and shorter hospital stays, preventive care is not likely to improve significantly in the near future. There are dangers in this for the health of all persons with disabilities. Consumers, rehabilitation professionals, family members, and other caregivers all need to heighten their monitoring of potentially life-threatening situations so that they are detected as soon as possible and do not develop into serious conditions. And persons with disabilities need to take charge of their health. As Brian advised based on his experiences:

- Find a balance of time with others and time alone

- Get creative and find some hobbies to keep your mind busy

- Keep your body in shape and work out

- Eat well

- Don't overdo

- Try to fix what's not working for you.

- Get into a support group

- Explore what's on the Internet and in books

- Get counseling and support when "feeling down and in a rut"

    Research evidence shows that surviving into middle age and older with a disability doesn't result from good health alone (e.g., Krause, DeVivo, Jackson, Pickelsimer & Broderick, 2004). While health behaviors are certainly important, it's an outcome of the blend of good health practices as well as the nature of the disability and its severity, one's emotional adjustment and health, and community integration.

For a variety of reasons, people make different lifestyle and personal choices. The individuals in this book with varying outcomes have handled issues with housing, transportation, employment, relationships, personal assistance and assistive technologies in different ways. Maggie and Brian come across as strivers, Ann and Linda as survivors. Then there are the casualties: Ken of an incurable disease, Butch of his outlook and family, and Jim of his expectations. Where Brian adopted an attitude that life is full of interesting challenges and opportunities, others focused on obstacles. Brian left his home for California whereas Butch did not seek independence from his family and remained in his parents' home. Maggie, Brian, Ann and Linda, and Jim did not like to be held back and found ways to win their battles and get out of their individual states of *stuck*.

Was there anything in their first interviews with me and in their personality profiles that offered clues to these outcomes? As mentioned earlier, individuals in this book completed the *Taylor-Johnson Temperament Analysis* (TJTA) and the *Defense Mechanism Inventory* in 1986. Here are the results (Jim, Ann and Linda did not complete the measures):

Butch. On the TJTA Butch responded that he felt nervous, depressed, inhibited, quiet, indifferent, hostile, and impulsive. He also scored high on submissiveness. His pattern of scores indicated emotional repression, which showed in the ways that he presented himself as a gruff individual, but actually had sensitive feelings that came through in the poetry he wrote and the rug that he made for his mother. He also showed that he had a tendency to turn anger inward and towards the self. Recall in Chapter Five that Chris had said to him, "Your biggest problem is *you*, sweetie" and recognized he needed a "different approach." Butch received Chris' lowest rating on "adaptive behavior."

Maggie. Her TJTA profile had high scores on the following traits: nervous, depressed, inhibited, indifferent, hostile and impulsive. Her ego defense mechanisms indicated active coping mechanisms. In particular, she deals with conflict by ascribing negative characteristics to it and then attacking the external frustrating object. Her running into obstacles in her path with her wheelchair is an example of how Maggie deals with frustration. Her speech therapist had rated her highest functioning in the area of adaptive behavior.

Of all the individuals in the book, Butch and Maggie had the highest scores on hostility and indifference. Whereas Butch had a profile of being submissive and quiet, Maggie had a dominant profile. Butch would withdraw; Maggie alienates others (recall her discussion about losing her job). Butch's profile suggests feelings of inferiority and inadequacy that led to him shutting off his deep, inner feelings as protection against hurt.

Brian. On the TJTA Brian reported being nervous, depressed, inhibited, sympathetic, and tolerant. He has a passive defense style and tends to be emotionally inhibited, finds it difficult to express warmth, and represses his affect. On the measures of personal capacities and functioning, he and his counselor (Chris) both gave him maximum scores on "adaptive behavior"

Chuck. According to his TJTA scores, Chuck is impulsive and hostile, with his hostility tending to be directed both towards himself and others. His profile suggests difficulty with remaining committed to a plan or goal.

Ken. Responses on the TJTA showed that Ken felt nervous, depressed, quiet, inhibited and submissive. His preferred ego defense style and means of dealing with conflict was to split off affect from content and repress the former. Rationalization and intellectualization are frequently observed in individuals with this style. He also scored high on being tolerant, sympathetic and self-disciplined, which are characteristics we typically associate with a caring and helpful individual. Ken's social work and rehabilitation counseling educational programs are line with this. In 1986, Chris had given Ken, like Brian, the highest possible score adaptive behavior."

There are many examples where the measures did pick up traits that were apparent in reading the individual narratives in this book. Counselor and therapist views of adaptive behavior were also accurate. Variability among individuals' personality traits and ways of managing their lifestyles are evident in every chapter.

What is quite striking is that everyone, except Chuck, scored very high in nervousness (anxiety) and depression in 1986. This was reported during a time when psychological services for persons with disabilities was not given a high priority — and the ensuing years have seen counseling services diminished even more. If there is one thing above all else that has been made clear by the individuals who have shared their experiences in this book it is that rehabilitation must become not only more focused on the person, but ready to assist that person through changing needs and preferences and confrontations with new disappointments and challenges.

Bereavement and stage models (discussed in Chapter Seven) present a "normal" pattern of psychological adjustment and developmental change, and are typically used as a yardstick against which to measure progress and *rehabilitation success*. As was discussed in Chapters Five and Seven, such standardized models are likely not the most effective means of addressing, and measuring, unique and individualized goals and accomplishments. Additionally, they may encourage a preoccupation with the person's limitations and level of distress. A better yardstick against which to measure *rehabilitation success* and *quality of life* may be the personal goals articulated by the individual and then tracking over time progress made in their attainment.

The same need exists in the use of measures of personality. While interesting information was obtained from the *Taylor-Johnson Temperament Analysis* (TJTA) and the *Defense Mechanism Inventory*, and psychometric assessment can be useful in developing intervention recommendations, there can be an inappropriate emphasis on psychopathology if a test has not been normed on individuals with disabilities. Profiles on some tests can be artificially elevated by reasonable concerns about physical functioning. For example, Elliott and Umlauf (1995), in a chapter that should be required reading for anyone using personality tests with individuals with disabilities, state:

> ...The lack of appropriate norms and comparison groups, as well as the insensitivity of cookbook approaches to item content contaminated by the physical concomitants of acquired disability, limits test interpretation and application. Not surprisingly, then, a personality profile might reveal that a respondent with a physical disability was preoccupied with physical sensations or ailments. Critics have justifiably argued for the development of separate norms so that meaningful and appropriate comparisons can be made with peers who have similar physical limitations' (p. 326).

Selective attention to certain traits and affective reactions combined with a frequent lack of cultural sensitivity has limited the relevance and appropriateness of many personality measures and has caused other problems experienced by people with disabilities to be ignored. For example, individuals would likely benefit from assistance in developing more resilience and resourcefulness in order to achieve a *disability experience* that is characterized by enhanced subjective well-being and quality of life, and not the mere minimization of disability. But this kind of intervention is very rare, making this an issue in need of attention.

Issues and trends in the field of rehabilitation in general, and assistive technology in particular, are discussed in the next chapter, along with recommendations for practice that have emerged from the ideas discussed up to this point.

Chapter Nine Footnotes:

[1] The U.S. government has two programs for people with physical or mental disabilities:

(1) Supplemental Security Income (SSI) gives persons with disabilities who are classified as poor a tax-free monthly check. States may add to this federal dollar amount. Additionally, the recipient receives health insurance through Medicaid.

(2) Social Security Disability Income (SSDI) is for individuals with a work history prior to having a disability.

Health insurance is provided through Medicare. In 1981, Congress enacted a measure which allows recipients to keep some of their benefits even if they go to work. Instead of losing benefits, cash payments are reduced by one dollar for every two dollars earned on a job. The Work Incentives Improvement Act (WIIA) further improves benefits for persons with disabilities who wish to work.

CHAPTER TEN

Still Living in the State of Stuck

Man is born free, yet everywhere he is in chains.
— JEAN-JACQUES ROUSSEAU

A rehabilitation engineer explained his view of the value of technology for people with disabilities as being similar to almost everyone's dependence on cars.

> I can get from my home to my job five miles away in a matter of minutes. Without my car, I couldn't live in that home and walk to work every day, in all seasons. My car extends my endurance and speed. Everyone uses technology for assistance.

The engineer's point is that technology provides tools we all use for assistance — devices to make tasks in our lives easier or more efficient. A non-disabled person chooses precisely the tool he or she thinks will be best suited to the task. The engineer, for example, probably considered various kinds of cars before he chose the best one for his commute. In the same way, a carpenter might choose between a hand saw and a power saw, depending on whether he was doing cabinet work or cutting huge sheets of plywood for a roof.

Since a great many persons equipped with the most appropriate assistive devices for their use can now lead more independent lives, more people with disabilities live in their communities, attend regular schools, and seek professional careers than ever before in our history. This is why we are hearing the plea to move away from the medical model of rehabilitation (with an emphasis on functional capability) to a social model (with an emphasis on inclusion and participation and support for this through universal design, legislation, and societal attitudes of acceptance as well as assistive devices, personal care assistants and service animals). This represents an evolution from a philosophy which emphasized that persons with disabilities should strive to be like non-disabled persons to a philosophy of empowerment, i.e., persons with disabilities have the right to be self-determining and to make their own choices about their lives and to achieve the quality of life each believes is personally best. Persons with disabilities want as much emphasis placed on their community (re)integration as on their physical

Figure 10-1:

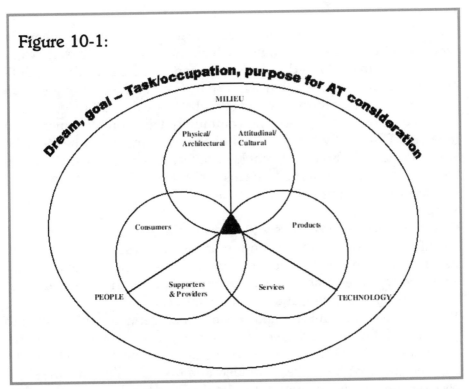

capabilities, creating as much need to change and accommodate the environment as equip the person.

TRENDS ON THE HORIZON

It often seems as if there are two opposing forces in rehabilitation today: (a) People with disabilities who want more comprehensive care, and (b) the realities of the need to contain costs and deliver services in the most cost-efficient manner possible. While it may be tempting to rely heavily on assistive technologies to help consumers become more independent in their functioning, more than ever, people with disabilities say they need and want comprehensive rehabilitation — especially rehabilitation that acknowledges and works with their feelings, moods, and attitudes.

As we move from a medical to a social model of rehabilitation, we can expect to see changes in how rehabilitation professionals work with consumers and deliver services. The chart in Figure 10-1 with its three interlocking circles represents the three broad MPT areas in which such changes will occur. Each circle is then divided into two often different, even opposing, halves. The area of overlap among the three circles is what will be necessary to achieve. The three circles are discussed in turn below.

Milieu

The physical/architectural and attitudinal/cultural environments in which services are provided and in which consumers will live and work will continue to be affected by legislation and changes in healthcare policies. Accessible transportation will need to be provided throughout an entire community (central city and suburbs). Assistive technology use in school, the home, workplace and community will all receive increasing attention. Disincentives to work will be minimized so that people who wish to work (like Brian) will not have to fear loss of benefits. There will also need to be improved means of ensuring adequate personal assistance for persons with disabilities.

People

Consumers. More consumers will receive college degrees and enter the workforce as professionals and managers. These consumers will demand accessible and reliable transportation services which allow for spontaneity. The education of consumers and caregivers will be done in part by distance learning and use of the Internet.

Providers. More healthcare and rehabilitation services will move into consumers' homes, and thanks to e-mail, pagers, voice mail, fax machines, and CD-ROM/DVD technology, personal contact can be supplemented with services provided at a distance. Yet, providers will become "user-centered" and not technology-centered. The quote below is from a vocational rehabilitation counselor who participated in person-centered assistive technology services and found the experience to be eye opening:

> In the past, locating and designing assistive technology devices for consumers has always been one sided. Since we were the ones paying for the bulk of expenses for the AT devices, we were always the ones to decide what a consumer needed. It was not unusual for us to find a certain device and then just order it hoping that the consumer would use it. This was the easy way out because we didn't have to put in extra time to make sure that the device was what the consumer wanted; we were just able to get something to fulfill our commitment. It's funny, that sounds so horrible but in honesty, we didn't give it a minute's notice. We just did what we needed to do and went on to consumer number two. The big problem that we were getting so frustrated with was that most of the consumers would only use the device for a little while and then abandon it. We just felt that they didn't need it any longer or didn't want to take the time to learn how to use it. It never occurred to us that it may not be a good fit for them because the device was never person- centered... I can't believe that I use to think I knew what AT device someone needed. If I don't have the consumer's input, how could I possibly know what they need?

Increasingly, consumers will "partner" with providers in product evaluation and selection. For professional and consumer partnerships to be effective, however, perspectives need to be openly shared and discussed. It will become increasingly important to be sensitive to cultural, ethnic and gender differences in assistive technology preferences and ways to present assistive technology options.

Assistive technology is a new field and one in which credentialing of practitioners is recent. Already, however, continuing professional development in assistive technology is being addressed as well as the education and training of new practitioners in the field. The delivery of instruction and continuing education will be accomplished as much by distance learning as in traditional classrooms.

Technology
Products. Technical advancements have increased the usability of technologies, improved components and materials, and generally contributed to enhanced consumer functional independence. There will be equal emphasis on making existing products lighter, more portable and streamlined and more affordable as on the design of new products. Modular or readily changeable equipment will be common. Computer proficiency will be increasingly important.

More than a decade ago, microprocessor-controlled wheelchair electronics were introduced. As computers and computerized components are used to develop more sophisticated assistive technologies, the additional complexity and cognitive load on the user will have to be dealt with much more adequately than has been done up to now. An array of options need to be developed for adequately training users and their caregivers in the operation and maintenance of these devices.

The concept of universal design (or "everyone fits") will gain wide acceptance in new products, housing and community facilities. Universal design ideally results in environments and products that are usable by everyone, and thus, their relevance to and usability by persons with disabilities is assumed and is as invisible as possible. Assistive technologies, on the other hand, tend to be products that are designed from the outset to enhance the functional capabilities of persons with disabilities. When an environment cannot be modified easily or cost-efficiently, when individuals live in dispersed neighborhoods, the least costly alternative may be a combination of universal design and assistive technology. The purpose of both universal design and assistive technology is to enable individuals to fully participate in all of life's activities regardless of capability or ability.

Medicine, too, will increasingly employ technology to enhance the lives of persons with spinal cord injuries (SCI). Technology has impacted bladder control and controlled voiding as well as fertility for men with complete SCI. Recently, many SCI centers have implemented specialized programs which use new technology (electroejaculation or vibratory stimulation) for assisted sperm retrieval with excellent results in terms of fertility. There are now many men who have fathered children post-SCI, something that few thought possible 20 years ago. For example, since beginning its program in 1996, the University of Rochester Medical Center has helped six couples achieve pregnancy. Recent research (e.g., Rintala, Herson, & Hudler-Hall, 1999) has confirmed that the parenting styles and effectiveness of persons with SCI is not essentially different from the general population.

Services. Rehabilitation professionals will face the need to inform a wide range of the public about the availability and benefits of assistive technology in ways that can reach them easily and in an understandable, personalized way. More information about specific devices will be available on the Web and the use of information technologies will proliferate for narrowing down product options and ordering devices.

Improvements must continue in the funding and availability of technologies. To keep the focus on the user of these products and services, providers will assess user preferences and priorities before selecting appropriate devices. Predispositions to the use of particular technologies, as well as the outcomes achieved from use, will also be assessed as the field moves more solidly towards evidence-based practices.

Assistive technology is an important field for the future. Measuring functional capability in different contexts and over time to demonstrate change in the capabilities of individuals will be very important. Measures need to be simple and straightforward and identify targeted goals in terms of what the consumer wants to achieve. For example, walking may be a rehabilitation goal, but not the individual's goal.

THE PROBLEM OF FUNDING

Funding for assistive technologies remains one of the biggest obstacles to matching the person with the most appropriate assistive technology, and it is a major topic at conferences and in the assistive technology literature. There is a growing gap between the haves and have-nots. Funding recommendations run the gamut from federal and state programs to service organization sponsorship and private fund-raising events. Some individuals take personal loans. Many individuals with disabilities feel as though they have been forced to return to the origin of the word handicap — "begging with cap in hand" — to get the equipment they need. Getting new or replacement devices has become so complicated and fraught with obstacles that the 1994 reauthorization of the Technology-Related Assistance for Individuals with Disabilities Act included a section on Protection and Advocacy Services (P&A), that is, legal assistance as a key element of assistive technology services. The 1998 Assistive Technology Act retained P&A services.

How Funding Occurs Now. Sixty to 65 percent of all assistive technologies are obtained through self-pay. But very few people with disabilities can easily afford to pay for high-tech or even low tech assistive devices on their own. And that's part of being stuck; not knowing where to go for assistance. While individuals obtain funding to pay for their devices from a variety of public and private sources, the majority of funding comes from the following sources. The information provided below was developed especially for this book by the Assistive Technology Law Center, Ithaca, NY:

1. **Private insurance plans** which include medical insurance (e.g., Blue Cross/Blue Shield) or accident insurance (e.g., automobile, home) will cover many devices needed to maintain the person's health and independence.

2. **Federal and state programs** may provide funding for devices when private insurance is not available or is no longer adequate.

    a. Special education is available for children with disabilities from birth to 21 years of age. Such children may receive devices through their school districts if the devices are necessary for the achievement of educational goals. The Individuals with Disabilities Education Act or IDEA requires each public school system in the U.S. to serve students with disabilities and give them a "free and appropriate" education.

    b. Vocational rehabilitation serves people with disabilities who have the potential for work. Federal/state vocational rehabilitation programs (described in Chapter Five) define the potential for work very broadly to include many types of activities beyond full-time competitive employment such as part-time, sheltered, and supported employment as well as homemaking Vocational rehabilitation services may assist people to transition from secondary education or pursue postsecondary programs or vocational training. If a device is determined to be necessary for employment, or becoming employable, then vocational rehabilitation services will pay for it. If a person is not seeking employment, and a device is necessary for a person's independence, the person may receive assistance from an independent living program or center.

c. Medicare, Part B serves persons 65 and older as well as those who have been receiving social security disability insurance benefits for a period of 24 months and persons with disabilities whose parents are disabled, retired or deceased. Medicare, Part B covers durable medical equipment and prosthetic devices that are determined to be "medically necessary."

d. Medicaid may pay for devices not covered by private insurance for those who meet financial criteria. As with Medicare, the device must be "medically necessary."

e. The Veterans Administration will pay for technologies considered part of a medical or rehabilitation program for veterans of the U.S. armed services.

f. Recipients of Supplemental Security Income (SSI) can put money aside for the purchase of work-related technologies under the PASS program (Plan to Achieve Self Support).

g. Workers' Compensation will cover devices for independent living and/or to return to the workplace for workers injured on the job. To be eligible, individuals must have received their disabilities while covered under an employer's policy (while on the job).

h. Many states have taken the fees collected from DUI and traffic violations and have established a fund that supports research, the provision of assistive technology, and so on to eligible state residents.

3. **Charitable sources** can assist persons with particular disabilities who work through organizations by or for people with that disability (for example, the United Cerebral Palsy Associations) to obtain equipment. Private organizations such as the Lion's Club, Kiwanis, etc. may support the cause of a person who needs devices for independence.

Community medical equipment and home health care dealers/providers are often very knowledgeable about payors for particular kinds of devices and many have an individual on staff who assists people in applying for funding. Also, each state presently has a Tech Act project that has been funded through the Assistive Technology Act. The state projects serve as information and referral sources. To locate any particular state project, contact the RESNA Technical Assistance Project at 703/524-6686. RESNA (Rehabilitation and Assistive Technology

Society of North America) is an interdisciplinary professional organization focused on assistive technology.

As technology use among persons with disabilities has become more widespread, and as technologies continue to become increasingly sophisticated, the demand for them and their share of the budget pie is rising. Funding sources are finding it increasingly difficult to process requests for technologies with their available budgets and must determine where the greatest number of consumers can get the most benefit for the least amount of money. As a result, responses to requests for funding are slower and slower in coming, the application process has become increasingly complex, and the criteria for eligibility to receive funding more difficult to meet. Today, many persons with disabilities with good budgeting skills are able to get along by putting together a funding package comprised of family assistance, government funding and support, living with friends, and so on. Those without such skills can become stuck.

For persons requiring an assistive device for the first time, and for those who need to replace old or worn-out equipment, a great deal of effort and time is required first in contacting a source for funds and then in waiting for approval or disapproval. Paradoxically, while assistive technologies offer persons with disabilities better and more frequent opportunities to pursue an active and independent lifestyle, difficulty in purchasing these technologies often restrains them or even drives them backward.

The Realities of Funding. When I inquired about new equipment in 1995, most of the individuals in this book said they did have some new replacement devices. Once the equipment was ordered, it was delivered relatively quickly, but often it took many months (and sometimes more than one attempt) to get the funding approved. Chuck's experience illustrates how frustrating it was for him to get the most appropriate assistive technology.

> I got a new wheelchair last week. My other one I had since 1983 and it had a lot of problems. Actually, there were problems from day one. When I first got it, there was a lot wrong that they had to readjust. Then I had a lot of little problems. It was a new model, a live and learn chair... for twelve years. I had to use reverse for a brake because it wouldn't stop by itself. It would have both fuses going trying to go down too steep a hill. Then when you got down you lost all control of it. Or if you were going up a ramp and you blew a fuse, you lost control of the chair because it would just go do whatever it wanted to do. I took a few dumps in that chair. They offered to put a brake in, but it wasn't anything I could use myself. I'd need somebody standing beside me.

The new one is a big improvement. When I let off on the control, it stops. And the turning radius is much better. But it's very sensitive. I have to watch my hand. If I don't watch it, I don't always know if I'm moving it. That's just something I have to get used to, you know, like going from a Volkswagen to a Corvette.

It took about 10 months from the time we ordered it because it was rejected by Medicare three times before it got approved. Once it got approved, and it cost over $13,000, it only took about 2 months to get here. But I don't have the proper leg rests yet. It's narrower than my other one and doesn't have a real high back. And the seat is a little harder. It has a metal piece in the back with leather over the part you sit on, that you put the cushion on. That's a little firmer, but it makes the chair a lot more stable. But I've got a red spot I have to watch. I don't know if it's because of the chair.

Many technologies remain expensive, and there is often no follow-up support to make the necessary adjustments for a good match of person and technology. Serious complications can arise from this lack of attention; for example, pressure sores, or *decubitus ulcers*, and other health-related conditions can result.

In March 1995 I asked Ken, the social worker who used a wheelchair, about his numerous personal experiences dealing with Medicare, Social Security, etc. I asked for his thoughts about what would happen to others in similar circumstances who are not as knowledgeable as he is. Based on his own experiences in New York State, he said:

If they are lucky enough to have a good doctor who will do the paperwork, and they have a good community health nurse, then that's who would do it. Otherwise you go without until the decubitus [pressure sore] gets so bad you go into the hospital. And that's more expensive because it's a four week hospital stay that involves surgery. But you have to factor in emotional strain on the person. So, you're stuck. And that's just one example. Other examples are... [W]hen they limit the amount of nurse's aide service you can receive, then you end up going to a nursing home of some type. Which, again, is more expensive. It's expensive and it takes away from people's individuality because they have to conform to that institutionalized system.

Now when it comes to getting equipment, I've always had good luck. Again, I can speak for myself, so that helps when it comes to dealing with medical suppliers — and I also have a good relationship with the supplier here, so they will push the paperwork for me. My doctor is willing to fill out all the paperwork needed. He doesn't have that many people in my condition, and that's why he's probably more willing to do it.

Every three years you can get a new wheelchair, and that's probably about how long most of them last. But again, if you don't have a good relationship with a medical supplier, if you aren't real vocal, you aren't going to get things. I know people who've had the same wheelchair for ten years and it's falling apart. They can't get a new one because they don't know how to work the system in order to get it.

I described to Ken the attempts that Chuck had made to get a new wheelchair (after twelve years) and asked why he thought Chuck's request for a new one was turned down three times.

Either the doctor didn't write the exact right thing — or sometimes they reject them because they figure if they reject them, then you may not need them and you won't reapply. That's what they do at Social Security. They routinely deny the case, about 80-85% on the first try, and then you have to apply again for a fair hearing and then you usually win. They deny it on the fact that if you're trying to get it illegally or whatever, and you don't qualify, more than likely you aren't going to bother with a fair hearing, reapply, and all that. One person I used to talk to who is an advocate for Social Security used to say that a couple of times she had to also tell them when they reapplied to reapply for funeral funds because they would be dead before they got Social Security. And, usually they were.

Now for people who can't speak as well for themselves, for example people with developmental disabilities, there can be a case manager involved. The case manager comes in to help with finances, getting the services they need and basically, pretty much do everything for the person. They don't have power of attorney, though. As it is, there's not enough case managers to go around, so the existing ones have unbelievable client loads.

I think it's going to get worse. A lot of choice will be lost for people on Medicaid with disabilities. There will be no housekeeping services any more.

In 1995 Ken anticipated reduced services in many areas. But, he said, there are some services that are so important, but already in such short supply, that it is difficult to imagine how things could get worse.

Have things gotten worse? As we read in Chapter Nine, getting new or replacement assistive devices in 2004 is costly, complex, and frustrating as a result. Maggie paid the $8,000 cost for her *Pathfinder* with her own funds so she could have it when she wanted it:

To have Medicare pay for it, I would have had to wait for the *Liberator* to wear out and confirmed to be non-repairable, and I didn't want to wait.

Ann and Linda are both waiting for new power wheelchairs that recline.

We were both fitted. However, Medicare is so slow, it might be a year before we get them.

More options need to be found for people with disabilities to obtain assistive technologies. Information on funding devices and getting training in their use needs to be made widely available on the Web and in various media.

OBTAINING ASSISTIVE TECHNOLOGIES IS AN ART AND A SCIENCE

As noted in Chapter Three, 6.2 million people used assistive devices in 1969. By 1990, more than 13 million people were using assistive devices, and the number of users continues to climb. Along with this growth, there have been many changes in making assistive technology devices and services more widely available:

- Professionals are now trained to understand and better match persons with assistive technology devices and services. Each state and U.S. territory has received funding through the Assistive Technology Act of 1998 to continue efforts, begun under the 1988 Tech Act, to inform its citizens of assistive technology devices and services. however, this legislation needs reauthorization, which had not occurred as of September 2004.

- In spite of more information being available, however, many professionals, teachers, parents, and consumers say they do not have the information or training they need to confidently consider options in assistive technologies. Much more education about assistive technology devices and services is needed. There must be more incentives for professionals to get this training, and it has to be affordable.

- There is a growing emphasis on outcomes measurement and credentialing of assistive technology professionals. A key aspect of outcomes measurement is providing evidence that shows particular consumer goals have been identified and then achieved. Outcome data will become increasingly essential in order to justify the need for assistive technology evaluation, provision, and training.

- It is now recognized that users of technologies have changing needs and preferences that require regular assessment to assure their assistive technologies are appropriate for them. When a technology is changed or added, it often requires other changes in the home or workplace, modifications to other technologies being used, or additional training for family and personal assistants.

- More attention is now being paid to the usability of devices (e.g., Richardson & Poulson, 1994). People select technologies based, first, on how well they satisfy functional needs and preferences, and then according to their attractiveness and appeal. If it meets the person's performance expectations and is easy and comfortable to use, then a good match of person and technology has been achieved.

Figure 10-2 diagrams this view of technology selection and use in a pyramid form similar to Maslow's motivational needs hierarchy (discussed in Chapter Seven). The diagram can be thought of as a usability hierarchy; lower-level criteria need to be met before one can be expected — or motivated — to move up the hierarchy. If lower-level needs are not met, the likely outcome is avoidance or non-use of the technology or dissatisfaction with using it.

There are additional complexities when equipping a person who has multiple disabilities with assistive devices, or equipping any individual with multiple devices that are each likely to have its own means of input, control and demands on the user due to multiple and overlapping hierarchies. With these overlapping hierarchies, it also becomes very important to consider issues arising from overequipping persons and problems from device overuse and cognitive strain. The coordinated management of multiple and complex devices will undoubtedly become a key rehabilitation goal in the near future.

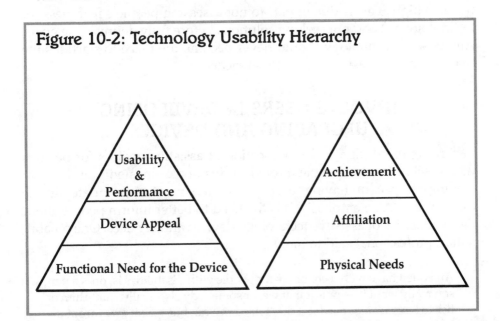

Figure 10-2: Technology Usability Hierarchy

Usability & Performance

Device Appeal

Functional Need for the Device

Achievement

Affiliation

Physical Needs

- Recognition in spreading the value of assistive technologies during hospitalization, for independent living in one's home, and for all community residential options. Yet there is also the understanding that individuals need to incorporate technologies into their routines in a way that makes the most sense for them and their significant others. For example, the use of family assistance rather than technology for a less important task may save physical energy for a more important task. Individuals need to achieve their own best blend of personal and technological assistance, as Brian described in Chapter Six.

- The perspective of the consumer is increasingly a primary focus. The potential technology user should drive the process of matching person and technology. Trial periods with devices should be available before final device selections are made, and people should be assessed and trained in the settings in which they will actually use their devices.

- Rehabilitation engineers need additional support in the human services they deliver. While educated for technical careers, they increasingly find themselves needing to provide psychosocial interventions. These highly motivated and relatively new additions to the comprehensive rehabilitation team merit increased attention to their unique roles.

Despite positive changes in the delivery of assistive technologies, the rate of technology non-use, inappropriate use, and abandonment remains high. This is due in part to not assessing people's readiness for technology use and not seeking solutions before fully defining the goals. An assistive technology should never become the place to start; it's the tool by which a desired outcome is reached.

INVOLVE USERS IN DEVELOPING UPGRADING AND DEVICES

Regarding the design and modification of assistive devices for persons with disabilities, the people quoted in this book repeatedly underscore the importance of having users select the most appropriate device for their use. Also emphasized is the need to better inform people about the availability of assistive technology devices and services. One rehabilitation professional said to me:

> An issue I have with technology for people with disabilities is, does a person really want it — or is it that we, or somebody else, really wants him or her to have it? Not need it. I don't need my car, but take it away from me

and I'll be very upset. But you can't want something you've never seen or heard of, so we need to expose people to the equipment so they can be informed consumers and make up their own minds about wanting it and using it.

Technology alone is rarely the answer to a person's enhanced quality of life. Assistive devices can help a person access more opportunities and exercise more options, but they require support services and training, attention to the person's personality, preferences, and capabilities and the characteristics of the milieu in which the device will be used. Rehabilitation professionals — counselors, psychologists, physicians, nurses, engineers, or occupational, physical, or speech therapists — must increase their focus on the emotional and social aspects of individuals' quality of life. Individuals with disabilities frequently have many unmet basic needs that require attention before assistive technologies should even be considered.

A major path to ensuring that devices address the tasks intended for them is getting users actively involved in the decision-making process. Involving consumers in the design and field-testing of prototypes of assistive devices helps assure that the devices will produce safe and reliable functional gain, that they are comfortable to use and aesthetically pleasing, and that self-esteem and quality of life are enhanced by their use. Chris, the OVR counselor with polio, advised: "Utilize the pool of users to try out new equipment and for their input, which can be considerably positive at times as far as the contribution of ideas."

The consumers profiled in this book realize the value of this practice and are willing to participate in prototyping devices:

Maggie: "People with disabilities should develop devices. I myself have suggestions for improvements if someone would just ask me."
Jim: "I think they should ask users more often what they see the uses being, not just to assume they're going to be helpful."
Ken: "There is a definite need for more prototyping. Let us have input into it because too many times we have stuff that's not appropriate."

Consumers are the ideal choice for developing and prototyping assistive technologies. There are many technically oriented consumers with disabilities who, like Maggie, are just waiting to be asked for their opinions. Consumers (and parents of young consumers) are naturally motivated and their involvement should be encouraged.

There is an additional benefit to consumer-driven design and testing of devices. Those involved early in the use of a new device —especially a "nonessential" one — serve as role models who encourage utilization of the technology by others. As Ken pointed out, "Many people might find devices less imposing if a peer was used as a model — to get the person interested." Peer modeling and support are valuable for presenting assistive technologies as options to individuals. Peer models also help others develop self-confidence, a positive identity, and a willingness to learn adaptive behaviors in general.

PEOPLE NEED SUPPORT FROM PEERS

Assistive devices are important enabling factors in independence and full community integration, and they can potentially equalize the capabilities of persons with and without disabilities. They can render a disability irrelevant or, at least, relegate it to a minor role. The view of a well-blended society where individuals from diverse background experiences and cultures live and work together often does not take into account the desire many individuals with disabilities have to belong to a peer group comprised of people who share and understand *disability experiences.*

Chris, the rehabilitation counselor with a disability from polio, is concerned that young people with disabilities do not have frequent opportunities, either inside or outside their inclusive educational settings, to talk with others with similar disabilities in order to share ideas and experiences. She believes that without such sharing, it is more difficult for them to establish a firm identity.

> ...When you're a needle in the haystack, it's very hard to find other needles... Today, people with disabilities don't meet enough people within their [cap]abilities. We need to build peer groups around rehabilitation programs that then get absorbed into the community.

But, as Jim's example illustrates, being with primarily non-disabled persons does not necessarily prevent mutual sharing — and contact with disabled peers does not guarantee it. A 31-year-old woman with cerebral palsy, who spent many years in an institution with others with similar disabilities, married a man with cerebral palsy (CP), and they are living independently. She highlighted the lack of information-sharing arising from being only with peers:

> Until a few months ago, I didn't know I had this [rheumatoid arthritis]. I thought every CP had this pain and that it was just a part of me, part of having CP. One night I asked my husband, "What do you do about the pain you're having?" And he said, "What pain?" I said, "The pain we all have... don't you know what I mean?" He said, "No." And that's the first I was aware my pain was different.

Chuck had mentioned that his rehabilitation occurred in a social vacuum. In a later interview he said, "We felt imprisoned. Whenever a quad came in for a checkup or something, we would ask what it's like on the outside."

A rehabilitation professional addressed the kind of social vacuum that can exist for individuals with cerebral palsy who live in group homes:

> You know, Marcia, I couldn't stand living in one of our residences. We are over-regulating people's lives. They're always working on some goal or another and staff have to be constantly documenting it and writing it down. The residents are exhausted. They haven't been taught ways to handle free time because they have no free time. And they don't know how to plan their own day because it's planned for them. Now I can understand the staff viewpoint — you have to do things for efficiency when you have 10 residents and two staff. But that's the same as what institutions do — work on efficiency rather than on individual needs.

As Chris said, "It's not good to have people only with others with the same disability. You can't win by keeping everyone in their own basket." She and Butch were in agreement on this. When I had asked Butch in 1991 if he had ever had any interest in joining a support group, he said:

> People really get tired of looking at other people in their shape. What's the fun of sitting around and talking to a bunch of people who know the exact same thing *you* know? Because they don't know any more, because they're not doing any more — and probably less.

While the individuals in this book acknowledged as many problems as benefits with inclusion, many advocated combining inclusive experiences with peer contact and support as an ideal solution to the weaknesses in each approach. In a 1991 conversation, Ken summarized this perspective:

> I think [inclusion has] left a lot of people isolated, but depending on the disability. A secondary support group on the side would allow for sharing of feelings and experiences. I think people would be isolated more if they weren't [in inclusive settings] and stayed alone in their own little group. They could be content but may get an institutionalized mentality. Without [inclusion] it's a lot harder to face the outside world. Rather than full, some people should consider partial [inclusion].

Some persons with cerebral palsy said they believe the combination of inclusion and peer contact would have greatly enhanced their own socialization efforts. For example, one woman said, "If I had been mainstreamed as a child, I'd be better adjusted and have more self-confidence now."

The lack of access to appropriate peers is a major gap in the rehabilitation system, which people have tried to fill on their own through such enterprises as the establishment of wheelchair sports teams and fellowships for persons with disabilities. Internet groups and chat rooms link individuals with shared interests and provide a wide array of information, but one must first have access to a computer. While these options help provide some peer contact, the gaps can hardly be said to be filled. At the beginning of the 21st century, it still remains difficult for a person with a disability to have a *disability experience* of achievement, belonging, and self-esteem.

IN SEARCH OF THE HUMAN TOUCH

The late sociologist Irving Zola (1984) pointed out, through examples of his own experiences with a disability, that no one, with or without a disability, is truly "independent." Rather than having independence as the goal of rehabilitation, it is better to provide individuals with the skills to:

- exercise self-directed choices

- manage their feelings

- request assistance with dignity and refuse it with diplomacy

- be assertive in job maintenance and advancement and in the establishment of new relationships

Then, individuals can ask for help without feeling they've lost self-control, individuality or independence, and they can better choose to use or not use devices.

Zola viewed technological assistance as the exchange of one dependency (human beings) for another (assistive devices). Regarding the use of devices, he asks: "Where does a healthy pursuit of independence end and a sad withering of human contact begin?" He cautions against objectifying care into a technical service, thereby objectifying the individuals receiving that service. He believes even "patronizing or infantilizing" care is preferable to assistance from robots or specially trained service animals because, as unacceptable or undesirable as these human interventions are, they at least reflect human qualities and maintain human contacts.

Brian, too, expressed why he believes robotics and service animals are not the answer for him. He used the example of feeding and said that some of his best times involved the close interactions that occurred then.

For many persons like Brian, life without assistance is not an option. Yet people cannot be blithely given a machine; people want and need people, interpersonal interaction and warmth.

There are positive and negative aspects to the use of assistive devices and personal assistance. While personal assistance is said to be the "key to employability of persons with physical disabilities" (Nosek, 1990), there are many cases where personal assistants have exploited consumers through theft or physical abuse (Ulicny, White, Bradford, & Mathews, 1990). Numerous examples were given in Chapter Seven of both the benefits and the challenges associated with assistive device use. The best course of action seems to be the prudent selection of the best of each. As Zola (1984) has stated, "It's not the quality of tasks we can perform without assistance, but the quality of life we can live with help..." (p. 123). Interdependence over independence. With or without technology.

GETTING QUALITY PERSONAL ASSISTANCE REMAINS PROBLEMATIC

People cannot perceive themselves as being in control — or be seen that way by others — if the first thing they have to face in the morning is a personal assistant who is late or does not arrive at all. The frustration this brings cannot be overstated. Professionals with disabilities want not only to arrive at work or a meeting on time, but to arrive looking good and ready to function in the role of a professional. For persons who are not working, but who want to lead an active life in the community, the frustration is just as great. And it is perhaps greatest of all for those, like Ann and Linda, who depend on personal assistance to avoid returning to a nursing home.

Consumers will increasingly employ personal assistants, not an agency. Consumers will want and need help in knowing how to interview, hire and train their caregivers. Brian has learned over the years through experience, and he shared his perspective with me:

> Living independently is like running a business. You need to approach it with a business head. What needs do you have? A person to talk to, help getting in and out of bed? To manage this for myself, I think about what needs to be done, the end goal, and then on the way to that how other needs can be met as well. It's a thinking process that I go through.

We have seen the struggles Ann and Linda have had with personal assistance, and Brian has had to hire and train many to care for him over the years. As these individuals age, their needs for personal assistance will likely increase.

Family Members and Their Needs are Often Overlooked

For many persons with disabilities, family members are crucial to the achievement of a satisfying quality of life. Yet, the process of trying to improve the quality of life for the person with a disability can be a very stressful one. At times, family members may feel anger and frustration toward the person with a disability and then feel guilty for having such feelings. Families frequently feel outnumbered by and distrustful of professionals, especially when their attempts to get equipment and other services are denied. When a person with a disability does receive new equipment, family members are typically the ones responsible for its maintenance and its transportation from one environment to another. Even though they know the individual best, and are also users of the technology, their opinions and ideas about equipment often go ignored. The frustration that builds may ultimately detract from their own quality of life.

The needs of family caregivers and the roles they assume require further study. More assistance needs to be given to them. When a family member has a disability, changes must be made in traditional roles, lifestyles, and expectations. These changes may affect the entire family for a lifetime. The adjustment process for both family members and persons with disabilities needs increased attention and persons with disabilities need to know they can receive help in adjusting to new stressors and disappointments in their lives.

PHYSICAL REHABILITATION IS 90% MENTAL REHABILITATION

Several people in this book wished they had received counseling to improve their self-image and self-confidence and to help them derive strategies for dealing with life's challenges. Butch acknowledged that there needs to be a heightened emphasis on the psychological aspects of rehabilitation when he said,

> People in this condition need mental rehabilitation more than anything else. Because that's 90% of physical rehabilitation. Rehabilitation doesn't want to face that 'cause it's too expensive. So you adapt. You develop coping mechanisms — and some of 'em, like drinking, are not good ones. If way back then they'd given us good coping mechanisms, a lot of problems could have been prevented.
>
> Early on, when you're totally receptive to learning somethin' and your mind wants to find out what all the ands, ifs, and buts are about — if they'd get your inhibitions out, have a psychotherapist come in to get

you talkin', get you adjusted to the thought of it. But once you get four or so years down the road, you're totally in a rut, stuck. If I'd been given a chance to hash out what was going on in my mind, things probably would've been a whole lot different for me.

This is very similar to Chuck's point in Chapter One:

I wish I'd had counseling regularly... on a fairly regular basis. I'm not sure what would've come out of it, but if you see someone enough, eventually you're going to say something. Try to bring things out, some of the anger, and things like that. That was something that was never done, and that anger just sits in there and grows.

Brian, too, acknowledged that, "I get stuck in a situation and I have to figure out how I'm going to get out of it," which for him can involve periodic counseling sessions from a community agency. But he has the perspective that counseling services for people with disabilities is not generally available and believes that for some issues peer support may even be a better choice (in actuality, most comprehensive rehabilitation programs today include supervised peer support programs):

I was talking to this guy Bill who collapsed in a field and is now paralyzed from the waist down. No one knows why. He needed so much to talk to me. That's one thing they don't have are counselors. They have Ph.D. shrinks to figure out meds but nothing like what I can offer. Which is information on how I got to where I am.

A person with a recent spinal cord injury reflected, "In rehab they handle your broken neck, but the broken neck isn't the problem. The paralysis is the problem. They don't confront the paralysis." And Jim lamented while he was still working at the insurance company that:

I know I do good work and get the job done like "normal" people, but yet I realize I'm different, that I'm handicapped. And it's frustrating, because I have devices and... I've had a lot of rehabilitation but not much counseling and we need more counseling to go with the devices.

Back in 1991 I had asked Ken what he thought about the need for counseling services in rehabilitation, he said:

Right now the emphasis is on getting people up to the highest level they can physically. They don't have the time right now to help people bring up their self-esteem. I think somewhere down the line, they may have to work on it. It's going to have to be mainly on an outpatient basis — they'll have to start the person as an inpatient, and then follow the person. Rehab will get better. It's continuously gotten better through the years and will continue to do so. I think the same thing with assistive devices. The focus of rehab should be on getting people to do as much as they can, and even more, on the person's sense of self-worth.

As Brian noted in Chapter Nine, counseling services need to be (re)incorporated into comprehensive rehabilitation programs. Individuals would like opportunities to discuss and work through feelings, attitudes, and fears that interfere with rehabilitation. And, as has been discussed, the identification and reformulation of goals needs to be a first step, and then the provision of the technologies, supports and emotional resources to achieve them. In this way, rehabilitation interventions are best accepted and adopted by the consumer.

Our *vital connections* develop and re-develop over time and when we don't feel connected to other people, a life role, and a goal, we feel stuck. The re-establishment of such connections is a primary goal for counseling services. Thus, counseling needs to be given a priority because it will ultimately save many dollars and pay for itself in helping persons who are depressed, who abuse substances, who need to develop new coping strategies and new relationships, and who need to come to terms with barriers to their own functioning, sense of connection and belonging, and motivation. Counseling specialists, trained to have an interactive, comprehensive and interdisciplinary approach to problem intervention, can — as Chris had once said to me — "look at the whole picture: pride, motivation, confidence, coping, one's outlook on life — all those elusive things." They can help people with disabilities resolve identity confusion and come to terms with and enhance their own unique circumstances. For some persons, this may mean developing a positive view of their differences. As Garris (1983) said:

> I mentally cringe when I hear people with disabilities say they are like everyone else — I am not and I know why. My life experiences have been quite different, the problems that I've had to solve have been different. It's little wonder that I'm different in so many ways. Viva.

"ONE MAY LEARN TO AMBULATE ON ARTIFICIAL LIMBS, BUT HAVE NOWHERE TO WALK"

In the late sixties — the era of Lyndon Johnson's Great Society — an essay on "Professional Antitherapy" (Kutner, 1969) had this to say about the passive-receptive role patients are expected to play throughout their rehabilitation:

On the one hand, the patient is taught how to get well again by means of specific techniques of muscle and habit training. On the other hand, this education is carried out in a social vacuum, divorced from the hurly-burly of daily life. The patient is taught generically useful habits but is kept from exercising them by a contrived context not remotely approaching the vicissitudes of life in open society. One may learn to ambulate on artificial limbs, but have nowhere to walk ... learn to speak, but have no one to communicate with or no drive to use this power to gain useful objectives (e.g., negotiating for a new apartment, arranging for transportation, joining a club or church, developing new friends) (pp. 177-8).

This essay appeared over thirty years ago, but the individuals who have shared their experiences in this book have all showed that it is still quite current. Several said that, in spite of such efforts as independent living services, the Americans with Disabilities Act, and their own accomplishments, they still feel inadequate, like marginal participants in society. They feel abandoned or betrayed by the system designed to help them.

Too many persons with disabilities in the U.S. have what Ken termed "a low-grade depression." For some, old friends have disappeared without new ones to take their place, or there has been a deliberate rejection of friends. Like Butch in the early years after his injury, they feel connected to no one, find little to hope for. They often have become emotionally inhibited or repressed. They are lonely and they believe that no one understands their feelings — or cares. Goals and motivation, potential, purpose, and meaning are elusive. They are in cycles of despair, and too many eventually commit suicide.

While some individuals cope by withdrawing, turning to alcohol and drugs, or developing chronic health problems, others cope through a "drive to survive" and set their sights on opportunities, not limitations. Just how any given individual's *disability experience* develops depends on the complex mix of details comprising the person's temperament, expectations, prior experiences and opportunities, and psychosocial environment. It also depends on aspects of the disability and the type and amount of rehabilitation and "empowering resources" (for example, assistive devices and vocational training) made available to the person.

In 1991, Butch said, "We need to change our own attitudes and those of society — have people and society blend better, them to us and us to them." The quality of life a disabled person is able to achieve is interactive and contextual. It is affected by the rehabilitation system's emphasis on its own maintenance rather than the provision of full and comprehensive rehabilitation that includes psychosocial interventions and training. It directly correlates to the importance placed on modifying individual functional limitations: the message to be compliant yet independent, to be yourself yet to emulate the "ideal," to see assistive devices as keys to new opportunities, but to keep expectations realistic. It is very much influenced by on-again, off-again legislation and by society's degree of tolerance at any given moment. It is tremendously impacted by the subtle message that machines and technology will provide a better life.

We are physically rehabilitating people — far beyond what has ever been possible before now. But what are we rehabilitating people into? It seems we need to keep asking that question until we can define "rehabilitation success" primarily in terms of the quality of life persons with disabilities can achieve, rather than the quality of care or quality of technology they may receive.

CONCLUSION: THE LIFE STORIES OF PEOPLE WITH DISABILITIES ARE LIFE STORIES OF US ALL

As useful as technologies are, we still do not know enough about how they affect the individuals who use them. This book was written to help fill this gap by describing the lives of people who use technologies to help them with critical tasks, as well as those who have tried and then abandoned or discarded them. It has advocated a "person first" perspective in order to ensure that technologies enhance individuals' quality of life.

When personal computers flooded the country in the 1980s and 1990s, they fueled dreams of possibility and of freedom from the more mundane aspects of life. In actuality, their widespread use has often isolated people and created highly stressful work environments.

Technology is ubiquitous. By many accounts, however, technological advances have not made us happier or our world better. We have remained a society modeled after the machine, where conformity, synchronicity, and predictability reign.

So, it seems, we are all stuck. We live in a society with many opportunities, but we increasingly have fewer freedoms within them. We are confused by social advances and retreats and sophisticated medical and technical achievements. Now that our jobs can be done by computers, our hearts kept going by pacemakers, our unhealthy organs replaced by those taken from someone else, we find ourselves wondering if we really need more and better technical advances. The cure for AIDS still evades our search, our air and water are badly polluted, and old diseases like cholera and tuberculosis are returning. All is not running as smoothly as the machine. Yet we have become less interdependent on people and more dependent on technology. Now we are thinking that we first need improvement in the basic things, like quality education, affordable health care, and housing.

We all frequently feel alienated from the systems designed to support and help us — that we're *living in a state of stuck*. We are all encouraged to be individuals, but pushed to do as we're told. All of us too often have no one to talk with, even if we can speak. Through it all, the machines and the computers keep rolling along.

Our quality of life is not always as we wish. Quality of life is not just the absence of poverty, pain, and other aspects of human suffering. It is not just extending the length of an individual's lifespan. It isn't about the prevention of dying, but the enhancement of living. It is not a matter only for social scientists and health care professionals. Quality of life is the sum total of the way we feel and think about ourselves, the environments we put ourselves into, the kinds of people we associate with, the systems and institutions with which we choose to become involved, the goals we have, the opportunities we are able to pursue, and the belief we have in our potential to effectively act on our environment. It is belonging, having purpose and meaning and having a vital connection to the world around us. While technology does provide many people with an important means of connecting, it is only one means.

No one wants technology to be taken away. But its use should come from choice, not from having it hurled relentlessly upon us. Too often, individuals with disabilities are excluded from decisions regarding assistive technologies and other matters which affect their lives. This exclusion perpetuates the belief that persons with disabilities are passive and incompetent. We need to understand how technology impacts society and its members, and how they can participate in this script. More than most persons, individuals with disabilities are very intimately involved with technologies. It is critical to ensure that these experiences are positive and enhancing, since the quality of these people's lives depends on them in very fundamental ways.

Since 1985, when I started looking at the influences on people's use of assistive technologies, there have been many improvements in the services and opportunities available to persons with disabilities from simple to complex technologies. Several pieces of legislation have been passed, all designed to enhance the quality of life for persons with disabilities, but other key pieces of legislation have been stalled. There is concern the ADA has been weakened and it is clear there is much that still needs to be done. Ken had summarized his view in 1995 as follows:

> There have been a lot of improvements since 1986. There's more housing, and more people can live in the community. Some of the technology has

gotten better, like lifts that allow a person to go from the bed to the bath, better wheelchairs, and improved safety devices — which have become important for living on your own. Outside the house, I don't see as much of a change, like with access to buildings and things like that. Just a slow change now that the ADA has gone through. You don't see many small businesses complying with it, and no one seems to be forcing them to comply. If there's no enforcement, it's going to fall through. Right now I don't see enforcement. If people don't follow the law, then it's not so great. And it hasn't changed attitudes. I'm afraid of apathy setting in.

The physical and attitudinal environments for people with disabilities need to continue to improve. In addition, there needs to be increased attention to the emotional aspects of disabilities, such as how to deal with loss and limitations, stress and disappointment, changes in one's *disability experience*, and how to meet needs for achievement and affiliation (as well as the basic needs for security and safety). The stress on individuals and their family members from repeated frustrations, disappointments, and battles needs to be better acknowledged and alleviated.

There is much concern about our collective quality of life in the 21st century. Perhaps there will come a time when technologies are so affordable that everyone can have everything they desire. Perhaps we will become a society in which all people — with or without disabilities — can live and work where they want, how they want, without fear and without having to fight for every little success. But meanwhile —

> *It is flying, irretrievable time is flying.*
> — VIRGIL, 2000 YEARS AGO, DURING THE FIRST CENTURY B.C.

Additional references:

Elliott, T.R. & Umlauf, R.L. (1995). Measurement of personality and psychopathology following acquired physical disability. In L.A. Cushman & M.J. Scherer (eds). *Psychological Assessment in Medical Rehabilitation* (pp. 325-358). Washington, DC: APA Books.

Krause, J.S., DeVivo, M., Jackson, A., Pickelsimer, E. & Broderick, L. (2004). Risk factors for mortality after spinal cord injury [abstract]. *Archives of Physical Medicine and Rehabilitation*, 85(8), E1.

APPENDIX A

Glossary

Adapted Devices/Adapted Equipment: a term used to refer to devices designed for the general population but are adapted in ways to be useful for people with disabilities (for example, eating utensils with built-up handles).

Acquired Disability: a disability acquired after the acquisition of language and after early socialization.

Activities of Daily Living (ADL): those tasks that a person performs during a typical day (grooming, bathing, getting into and out of bed or a chair, etc.). Instrumental activities of daily living (IADL) include: doing household chores, necessary business, shopping, and getting around for other purposes.

Advocacy Services: Service provided to assist individuals with disabilities and their family members, guardians, advocates, and authorized representatives in accessing assistive technology devices and assistive technology services (AT Act of 1998).

Assistive Technology

Device: Initially defined in the "Technology-Related Assistance of Individuals with Disabilities Act of 1988" (P.L. 100-407): "any item, piece of equipment, or product system, whether acquired commercially off the shelf, modified, or customized, that is used to increase, maintain, or improve functional capabilities of individuals with disabilities." Such devices can be low-tech (mechanical) or high-tech (electromechanical or computerized) and may compensate for sensory and functional losses by providing the means to move (e.g., wheelchairs, lifts), speak (e.g., communication devices), read (e.g., screen readers on computers for persons who are blind), hear (e.g., vibrotactile aids), or manage self-care tasks (e.g., automatic feeders, environmental control systems).

Service: initially defined in the "Technology-Related Assistance of Individuals with Disabilities Act of 1988" (P.L. 100-407): "any service that directly assists an individual with a disability in the selection, acquisition, or use of an assistive technology device."

Capacity Building and Advocacy Activities: According to the AT Act of 1998, efforts that empower people with disabilities to achieve greater independence, productivity, and inclusion in the community and workplace. These may be achieved through changes in laws, policies, and organizational structures or through facilitating and increasing access to, provision of, and funding for, assistive technology.

Communication Devices

AAC: Augmentative and Alternative Communication devices ("aug comm devices"): technologies and techniques. AAC devices range from word boards to computer based devices with voice output.

Word-board: a stiff, flat surface that contains the letters of the alphabet, numbers 0-9, and perhaps many key phrases such as 'thank you,' 'I want,' and so on. It is small and light enough to hold in one's lap. The user of a wordboard communicates by pointing to the board to spell out words.

Congenital Disability: a disability present before, during or immediately after birth.

Durable Medical Equipment (DME): As defined in the Medicare statute, DME is equipment that is expected to last for a substantial period of time, is subject to repeated use and not consumed by this use, is not needed by an individual in absence of a medical need, and is appropriate for use in the home.

Environmental Control Unit (ECU) or Electronic Aid to Daily Living (EADL): activates a variety of household appliances such as a coffee maker, TV, radio, lights, automatic dialing telephones, and intercoms through a variety of alternative access methods, such as switch or voice access. EADLs include a range of systems from simple reachers or sticks to computers and voice-activated electronic systems.

Independent Living: a philosophy advocating self-directed choice and the ability to exercise as many free choices as possible.

Information Technology: Information technology includes any product used to acquire, store, manipulate, or transmit information, such as computers, multimedia, telecommunications, copy machines, and the Internet.

Orthotic Devices: used to provide support for a weak part of the body (e.g., braces).

Personal Assistance: Care provided by individuals to help persons with disabilities with ADL and other activities. May be provided by family members, paid individuals, etc.

Prosthetic Devices: replace or substitute a part of the body (like arms and legs).

Rehabilitation: The working definition of "rehabilitation" used by most professionals in the field emphasizes the restoration of a person's physical, sensory, mental, emotional, social, vocational, and recreational capacities so the person can be as autonomous as possible and will be able to pursue an independent non-institutional lifestyle.

Social Security Benefits: Social security benefits for individuals with disabilities include: (1) **Social Security Disability Insurance** (SSDI) and (2) **Supplemental Security Income (SSI)**. Individuals may receive benefits from either or both programs, depending on their work history, age, and financial resources. See individual listings under these terms for more information about each program.

> **Social Security Disability Insurance (SSDI):** A federal program in the Social Security Administration providing monthly benefits to disabled workers and their dependents. A person builds protection through employment covered under Social Security (compulsory tax on earnings). The disability definition is an inability to engage in substantial gainful activity

because of any medically determinable permanent physical or mental impairment. Later amendments required that a person have a disability for at least five months in order to be eligible for SSDI.

Supplemental Security Income (SSI): The federally-administered Supplemental Security Income program provides income support to people 65 and over, as well as blind or disabled adults and children who have little or no income or other financial resources. In order to be considered disabled for SSI, an adult must be unable to engage in any substantial gainful activity by reason of a medically determinable physical or mental impairment that is expected to result in death or last for a continuous period of at least 12 months. Blindness is defined as 20/200 or less vision in the better eye with the use of correcting lenses, or with tunnel vision of 20 degrees or less. Children who have a physical or mental impairment which results in marked or severe functional limitations are eligible for SSI.

Switches and Switch Software: Switches offer ways to provide input to a computer when a more direct access method, such as a standard keyboard or mouse, is not possible. Switches come in various sizes, shapes, colors, methods of activation, and placement options. An interface device and software are usually required to connect the switch to the computer and interpret the operation of the switch. Some software programs have been developed specifically for use with a switch and can employ on-screen scanning. With on-screen scanning, the computer highlights (either by sound, visual cue, or both) options available to a user about what action he or she wants the computer to take. Using these specialized products, when a visual or auditory prompt indicates a desired keyboard or mouse function, the user activates the switch and the desired function occurs. [Source: Computer and Web Resources for People with Disabilities, Alliance for Technology Access, 3rd Edition, 2000].

Switch Mount. A device that allows a switch to be mounted in a variety of positions. A switch mount might be attached to a wheelchair and positioned to allow easy activation of the switch. The switch mount may be positioned at the head, knee, chin, foot, elbow, or other switch site.

Trackballs. A trackball looks like an upside-down mouse, with a movable ball on top of a stationary base. The ball can be rotated with a pointing device or hand.

[The Arizona Technology Access Program (AzTAP) web site has a glossary containing many computer-related terms: http://www.nau.edu/ihd/aztap/atinaz/glossary.html]

Universal Design: Under the AT Act of 1998, "universal design" means a concept or philosophy for designing and delivering products and services that are usable by people with the widest possible range of functional capabilities. Examples of universally designed environments include buildings with ramps, curb cuts, and automatic doors.

Vocational Rehabilitation: This refers to programs conducted by state Vocational Rehabilitation agencies operating under the Rehabilitation Act of 1973 to provide or arrange for a wide array of training, educational, medical, and other services individualized to the needs of persons with disabilities. The services are intended to help these persons acquire, reacquire, or maintain gainful employment. Most of the funding is provided by the federal government. Public Law 102-569, the *Rehabilitation Act Amendments of 1992*, increased access to assistive technology.

Word Prediction Programs: Word prediction programs enable the user to select a desired word from an on-screen list located in the prediction window. This list, generated by the computer, predicts words from the first one or two letters typed by the user. The word may then be selected from the list and inserted into the text by typing a number, clicking the mouse, or scanning with a switch.

APPENDIX B

Checklists for AT Evaluation and Selection

This appendix contains portions of a workbook produced and used by peer mentors sponsored by the Regional Center for Independent Living (Rochester, NY). It is based on the author's Matching Person & Technology assessment process (described in Chapter Eight).

Introduction

This Appendix is dedicated to the memory of Andrea Levy, MSW, who co-edited the original workbook and died February, 1999 from complications associated with muscular dystrophy.

In addition to Andrea Levy, the original workbook was developed through the collaborative efforts of: Lynne Sebring; William D. Heerkens; Dr. Marcia Scherer (Consultant and Board Member), and the experiences of mentors and consumers.

The peer mentoring process used by the Regional Center for Independent Living focused on the Matching Person and Technology (MPT) Model and self-assessment tools [http://members.aol.com/IMPT97/MPT.html] to help potential users of assistive technologies examine their preferences and expectations, family and environmental influences, economic factors, and training needs.

Responses to the items in the MPT assessments assist both consumer and service provider in making choices best suited to the consumer's needs. In many cases, correct choices help avoid the frustration caused by technology that is not compatible with the preferences, personality, and environment of the person.

As a consumer and potential assistive technology user, important questions need to be answered in order to obtain the assistive technology that will really further your abilities. Knowing who you are, what you need, and why will qualify you to be the expert. You can explain your wants and needs to others more easily and effectively. A better sense of self allows you to look outward with confidence to find choices. Choice is power. This power directs you to move forward and plan strategies based on those available choices and your expectations. Purposely setting goals keeps you moving forward rather than focusing on weaknesses and fears. This will occur when you practice self-determination and self-advocacy.

It is important to think about the resources you already have and identify what resources you still need. It will be helpful to do some self-examination of your goals, then your ideas for ways to achieve those goals. **A form follows to help in this process. It is called "Worksheet for Matching Person and Technology" and it is the first form in the MPT assessment process.** As you use this form, it is important that you focus on your current feelings and attitudes. Fill out the form in two steps:

- Write down your initial goals and include possible alternative goals

- Determine what would help you reach these goals

Once this is done, you will be ready to identify an action plan to address your goals and proposed interventions. You should commit to writing out and developing your strategies and action plans. Experience has shown that plans that are only talked about are not carried out as often as written plans. Written plans also can provide a reason for further actions such as funding or training, etc.

WORKSHEET FOR MATCHING PERSON AND TECHNOLOGY

In which of the following areas do you have difficulty?
(Fill in the areas that apply)

Speech and Communicating with Others:

_____

_____

_____

Goals:

_____

_____

What would help?

_____

_____

_____

Mobility:

_____

_____

_____

Goals:

_____

_____

_____

What would help?

_____

_____

_____

WORKSHEET FOR MATCHING PERSON AND TECHNOLOGY

In which of the following areas do you have difficulty?
(Fill in the areas that apply)

Eyesight:

_____

_____

_____

Goals:

_____

_____

_____

What would help?

_____

_____

_____

Hearing:

_____

_____

_____

Goals:

_____

_____

_____

What would help?

_____

_____

_____

WORKSHEET FOR MATCHING PERSON AND TECHNOLOGY

In which of the following areas do you have difficulty?
(Fill in the areas that apply)

Reading/Writing:

_____

_____

_____

Goals:

_____

_____

_____

What would help?

_____

_____

_____

Household Activities:

_____

_____

_____

Goals:

_____

_____

_____

What would help?

_____

_____

_____

WORKSHEET FOR MATCHING PERSON AND TECHNOLOGY

In which of the following areas do you have difficulty?
(Fill in the areas that apply)

Self Care:

_____

_____

_____

Goals:

_____

_____

_____

What would help?

_____

_____

_____

Social and Recreational Activities:

_____

_____

_____

Goals:

_____

_____

_____

What would help?

_____

_____

_____

On the next two pages are charts for short-term and long-term goals, attempts toward achieving the goals, and results. Transfer the ideas you write on to them to the *Worksheet for Matching Person and Technology* under "Goals" and "What would help."

Purposely setting realistic goals is a tool to keep you moving forward, even if one step is simply making a phone call for information. Any challenge is an opportunity to practice assertiveness through self-advocacy and self-determination.

Figuring out a strategy based on your goals and the choices available requires that you learn all you can. **Keep track of experiences and contacts you make. This record, too, will serve your memory and give you confidence.**

Periodic reviews of this knowledge may be helpful to meet realistic goals.

SHORT-TERM GOALS

DATE NOW	WHAT YOU WANT TO ACCOMPLISH	BY WHEN	WHAT WAS ACCOMPLISHED	DATE DONE

LONG-TERM GOALS

DATE NOW	WHAT YOU WANT TO ACCOMPLISH	BY WHEN	WHAT WAS ACCOMPLISHED	DATE DONE

SELECTING ASSISTIVE TECHNOLOGY (AT) DEVICES AND SERVICES

For persons about to select an AT for the first time, and for those who need to replace an old or worn-out one, a great deal of effort and time is required to find the most appropriate one. Your responses to the questions* that follow will assist both you (as consumer and technology user) and the service provider in making choices best suited to your needs. In many cases, correct choices help avoid the frustration caused by technology that is not compatible with your preferences and environments.

We came up with these questions because we know how hard it is to figure out what questions to ask and how easy it is to forget what we do wish to ask. The questions are divided into sections as examples for you to have handy when you are talking to rehabilitation professionals and assistive technology providers. The answers to these questions can also serve as important information to share with rehabilitation professionals and assistive technology providers as you work toward narrowing your device choices.

The checklists are divided into the following sections:

1. Characteristics, preferences, and resources of the person who will use the device:
   - service preferences and needs
   - AT preferences and needs

2. Characteristics and requirements of the milieu or environments of use.

3. Characteristics of the AT itself:
   - performance
   - maintenance
   - selection
   - purchasing
   - training

Each question has two boxes. The first is to indicate how important this particular question is for you, for this device. The other box is to rank how well this question is addressed. You can use any rating system you prefer, but here are options:

QUICK OPTION

Check the boxes that are most important to you BEFORE you go to see competing products. Make photocopies of each page after you check the important boxes so that you have a fresh set to use for rating each competing product. Be sure to label each page with the name of the particular device. When you

Footnote:
* Questions are compiled from (1) Living in the State of Stuck: How Technology Impacts the Lives of People with Disabilities, by Marcia J. Scherer, Brookline Books, (2) Evaluating, Selecting, and Using Appropriate Assistive Technology, by Jan C. Galvin & Marcia J. Scherer, Aspen Publishers, 1996, (3) New York State Office of the Advocate for Persons with Disabilities/TRAID brochures, and (4) mentors' experiences.

Example:
[x]

evaluate that product, put check marks in the boxes as you review each question. A question mark can indicate those questions where more information is needed. Use one of your photocopies for evaluating the next product so that you have a fresh start. When you are done looking at products, compare each one as far as how many boxes you checked as being important also have check marks for meeting that condition. The product with the most checks wins!

THOROUGH OPTION

Use the following scale:

IMPORTANCE:	PRODUCT SATISFIES CONDITION:
3 = very	3 = very
2 = moderately	2 = moderately
1 = somewhat	1 = somewhat

First put a number inside each box according to **how important that criteria is** to you BEFORE you go to compare competing products. Make photocopies of each page after you rate the importance of various questions so that you have a fresh set to use for rating each competing product. Be sure to label each page with the name of the particular device. Then, as you evaluate a product, write the number inside the box as far as **how well the product satisfies that condition**. Use one of your photocopies for evaluating the next product. When you are done looking at products, multiply the **importance** score you gave each condition by the number you gave for how well it **satisfies that condition**. Total these scores for each page, then add the page totals together for a grand total. Compare the grand totals for each competing product. The one with the highest score wins!

Example: Product A

Importance		Satisfies Condition	Total
3	X	2	= 6
1	X	3	= 3
(blank)	X	3	= 0
			Score = 9

Questions to Ask about Characteristics and Resources of the Person Regarding Service Preferences and Needs

---

NAME OF DEVICE: _____

Importance	Rating	
❑	❑	Does the service provider come to the home, school, or place of work to provide evaluations or services; or if not, are the service provider's hours and site accessible?
❑	❑	Did the service provider treat me with courtesy and respect?
❑	❑	Did the service provider indicate that we will work together and share information?
❑	❑	Did the service provider really hear what I said?
❑	❑	Have I informed the service provider clearly what my expectations and needs are?
❑	❑	Will I be actively involved in the selection process of my device(s)?
❑	❑	Are the services comprehensive from my initial assessment to follow-up?
❑	❑	If I need multiple services, will they be accomplished?
❑	❑	Will everything I'm getting (product, training, services) be integrated?
❑	❑	Does the service provider offer a team approach with multiple specialists? Will I have to coordinate services and providers?
❑	❑	Is there a duplication in services or products with any of my choices?
❑	❑	Can the service provider adapt to my changing needs?

NOTES: _____

_____

_____

_____

_____

_____

Questions to ask about Characteristics and Resources of the Person Regarding Service Preferences and Needs (continued)

Importance	Rating	
❏	❏	Is the service provider and/or staff who does evaluations knowledgeable, credentialed, and skilled?
❏	❏	Does the provider keep up with the latest developments and approaches?
❏	❏	Does the service provider provide an adequate range of services to meet all of my needs?
❏	❏	Have I compared service providers costs like I compared products?
❏	❏	Did the service provider apply pressure to buy right away or become impatient with my questions?
❏	❏	Does the service provider expect a commitment from me and can I meet it?
❏	❏	Can I afford the fees involved with the service?
❏	❏	Will I have coverage for training, maintenance, and/or service?
❏	❏	Does the service provider accept third-party payments such as Medicaid, Medicare, or private insurance?
❏	❏	If not, can other funding or payment schedules be arranged?
❏	❏	Will the service provider wait until a third party pays, or is payment expected at the time of service?
❏	❏	If the service provider expects me to pay up front, did I check with the third-party payor to learn if and when I will be reimbursed for all or part of the cost?

NOTES: _____

_____

_____

_____

_____

_____

_____

Questions to Ask about Characteristics and Resources of the Person Regarding AT Preferences and Needs

---

NAME OF DEVICE: _____

Importance	Rating	
❏	❏	Will this kind of device meet my demands?
❏	❏	Does it fit with what I learned from the *Matching Person & Technology* process?
❏	❏	Can I manage using this kind of device as independently as I want?
❏	❏	Is the size and weight of this kind of device manageable?
❏	❏	Will I feel in control of this kind of device?
❏	❏	Can I answer honestly that I am comfortable about using this kind of device?
❏	❏	Will I actually use the device, or is it apt to go unused?
❏	❏	Do I really need this device, or do I just *think* I need it?
❏	❏	Have I considered low-tech and other alternatives?

NOTES: _____

_____

_____

_____

_____

_____

Questions to Ask about Characteristics and Requirements of the Milieu or Environments of Use

NAME OF DEVICE:_____

Importance	Rating	
❏	❏	Will this device meet my needs in various situations and environments?
❏	❏	Do I need special features or parts because of the weather conditions in my area?
❏	❏	Do I need special features or parts because of the geography in my area?
❏	❏	Does the device have the stability I need in a variety of situations and environments?
❏	❏	Does the device have the durability I need in a variety of situations and environments?
❏	❏	Do I need to make changes in my environments to accommodate my use of this device?
❏	❏	If I need assistance to use this device, will it be available?
❏	❏	Will the desired assistance be available in each environment?

NOTES: _____

_____

_____

_____

_____

Questions to Ask about an AT's Performance

NAME OF DEVICE: _____

Importance	Rating	
❏	❏	Does this device do what I want it to do?
❏	❏	Have I seen it demonstrated?
❏	❏	Does it require some skills or capabilities I don't have?
❏	❏	Does the device require assistance that is not easily available to me?
❏	❏	Will this device meet the needs of my various situations and environments?
❏	❏	Is the size and weight of the device manageable?
❏	❏	Is there any chance of this product being discontinued in the fairly near future?
❏	❏	Could it be adapted if there are changes in my functional abilities, activities, and/or size?
❏	❏	Is the device durable?
❏	❏	Is it comfortable to use?
❏	❏	Does it fit in my car or van for easy transport?
❏	❏	Does the device have the stability I need in a variety of situations and environments?
❏	❏	Are the knobs, switches, straps, etc. accessible and easy for me (or caregiver, personal assistant) to use?
❏	❏	Are there extra features to make the product more versatile?
❏	❏	Are there extra features that I'll never use?
❏	❏	Are adaptations or additional parts necessary for this device?

NOTES: _____

_____

_____

_____

_____

_____

Questions to Ask about an AT's Maintenance

NAME OF DEVICE: _____

Importance	Rating	
❏	❏	Do I adequately understand the technical assistance for the product?
❏	❏	Will I have access to and information about repair and maintenance of the device?
❏	❏	Can I maintain the device myself?
❏	❏	Do I understand the maintenance schedule of the device?
❏	❏	Is customer service provided for the device?
❏	❏	Are repairs and parts available locally?
❏	❏	Is the average turnaround time for repairs reasonable?
❏	❏	Can the product be serviced at my home?
❏	❏	Do the service providers have loaners available if doing without is a problem?
❏	❏	Does the manufacturer offer a warranty?
❏	❏	Does the manufacturer's warranty give the coverage I need? (What limitations are there? Are there specific conditions of coverage? Are there hidden costs?)
❏	❏	Does the store or vendor offer a warranty (in addition to the manufacturer's warranty) on the device?
❏	❏	Does the store or vendor warranty give the coverage I need, for the length of time I want?
❏	❏	If I need an extended warranty, is it available, and can I afford it?
❏	❏	If the device needs assembly, is there someone who will do it?
❏	❏	Does the manufacturer and/or the vendor offer support services after the sale?

NOTES: _____

_____

_____

_____

Questions to Ask about Your AT Selection

NAME OF DEVICE: _____

Importance	Rating	
❏	❏	Have I looked the product over carefully?
❏	❏	Can I try the device before making a commitment to it?
❏	❏	Are there other people in my area who use the same device or a similar one?
❏	❏	Can I talk with someone who has used a similar device?
❏	❏	Have I acted on impulse, or have I thought this selection through?
❏	❏	Is the provider/supplier accessible for me?
❏	❏	Are store personnel readily available to me?
❏	❏	Are store personnel and salespeople courteous and respectful?
❏	❏	Was the salesperson easy to talk to and knowledgeable?
❏	❏	Did the salesperson of the device apply pressure to buy right away or become impatient with my questions?
❏	❏	Were answers vague or misleading?
❏	❏	Did the salesperson listen to what I said?
		Does the business provide the four "Cs":
❏	❏	Convenience?
❏	❏	Choice?
❏	❏	Continuity and reliability?
❏	❏	Courteous and prompt service delivery?
❏	❏	Have I checked with the Fair Business Council about the reputation of the business?

NOTES: _____

_____

_____

_____

Questions to Ask about AT Purchasing

NAME OF DEVICE: _____

Importance	Rating	
❑	❑	Is the same device I tried the one I am going to get?
❑	❑	Can I afford the device that I am interested in?
❑	❑	Do I have funding for this particular assistive technology?
❑	❑	Can I justify the funding of this device?
❑	❑	Are there additional costs for necessary add-ons?
❑	❑	Can I trade in the product or upgrade it at a later date?
❑	❑	Is the product in stock, or if ordered, will I get it when I want it?
❑	❑	Does the vendor know the product well?
❑	❑	Are my needs going to change from the time I order the device to the time when I get it?
❑	❑	Have I shopped around for the best device?
❑	❑	Have I shopped around for the best price?
❑	❑	Have I thoroughly read the warranty and sales contract agreements to check for:
❑	❑	Limitations?
❑	❑	Conditions of coverage?
❑	❑	Hidden costs?

NOTES: _____

_____

_____

_____

Questions to Ask about Training

NAME OF DEVICE: _____

Importance	Rating	
❑	❑	Do I need training to use this device optimally?
❑	❑	Is training available from people in my family or social network?
❑	❑	Can I have training from professionals if I want it?
❑	❑	If training is available, can I afford the cost?
❑	❑	Can the training take place in my home, and if not, can I arrange to get where it is?
❑	❑	Will third-party funding cover training costs?
❑	❑	Will training time be limited?
❑	❑	Will ongoing training be available?
❑	❑	Will training take place using my own piece of assistive technology?
❑	❑	Will training occur within a reasonable time of delivery of the device?
❑	❑	Will the training source offer support services after the training (for follow-ups and availability if questions arise after)?
❑	❑	Can I complete training in a reasonable amount of time?

NOTES: _____

_____

_____

_____

APPENDIX C

Resources

A representative but not comprehensive sample of key resources for obtaining further information on the topics in this book.

U.S. Organizations Focused on Assistive Technology

Alliance for Technology Access
2175 E. Francisco Blvd. Suite L
San Rafael, CA 94901-5523
Voice: (415) 455-4575
TTY: (415) 455-0491
Fax: (415) 455-0654
http://www.ataccess.org

RESNA (Rehabilitation Engineering and Assistive Technology Society of North America)
1700 North Moore Street, Suite 1540
Arlington, VA 22209-1903
Phone: 703-524-6686
Fax: 703-524-6630
TTY: 703-524-6639
http://www.resna.org

U.S. Organizations Serving Persons with Spinal Cord Injuries or Cerebral Palsy

National Spinal Cord Injury Association (there are local chapters)
Helpline (800) 962-9629
8701 Georgia Ave., Suite 500
Silver Spring, Maryland 20910
Phone (301) 588-6959
Fax (301) 588-9414
http://www.spinalcord.org

National Spinal Cord Injury Hotline
Paralyzed Veterans of America
801 Eighteenth St. NW
Washington, DC 20006-3517
Tel: 1-800-526-3456
http://www.pva.org

United Cerebral Palsy (there are local chapters)
1660 L Street, NW, Suite 700
Washington, DC 20036
Tel: 1-800-872-5827
Fax: 1-202-776-0414
http://www.ucpa.org

Web Sites Focused on Assistive Technology U.S.

ABLEDATA. This site is a national database of information on thousands of products that are available for people with disabilities. http://www.abledata.com/

Alliance for Technology Access. A national network of community based resource organizations to provide information and support to increase the access and use of assistive technology. http://www.ataccess.org

Assistivetech.net. This National Assistive Technology Internet Site provides up-to-date, thorough information on assistive technology devices and services, adaptive environments, and community resources. Users can search for AT devices by function or activity, keyword, vendor or product type. http://www.assistivetech.net/

Assistive Technology Data Collection Project: An InfoUse Site. Provides links to AT-Related Government Agencies, AT-Related Organizations, Disability Statistics Agencies/Organizations, and Other Disability-Related Organizations. http://www.infouse.com/atdata/links.html

Assistive Technology Partners. A compilation of services, projects, activities, and research dedicated to enhancing access to assistive technology at home, school, work and play for individuals with disabilities, their families, employers, and professionals providing services. http://www.uchsc.edu/atp/aboutatp.htm

Consortium for Assistive Technology Outcomes Research. Focused on improving measurement science for AT, reducing barriers to the use of AT outcome measures, and understanding the processes for AT adoption and abandonment. http://www.atoutcomes.com

DisabilityInfo.gov. The site organizes information and issues concerning disabilities into nine categories, listed as color-coded tabs at the top of every page. Simply select the tab of your desired category, and links related to that topic will appear on the left. http://www.disabilityInfo.gov

Disability Statistics. An Online Resource for U.S. Disability Statistics by the Rehabilitation Research and Training Center on Disability Demographics and Statistics at Cornell University. http://www.ilr.cornell.edu/ped/DisabilityStatistics/index.cfm

Do-It (Disabilities, Opportunities, Internetworking and Technology). Do-It provides resources on education, technology, accessibility, funding, and more. <http://www.washington.edu/doit>

EASI (Equal Access to Software and Information). EASI provides workshops, distance learning, webcasts, and other training on information technology. EASI's mission is to serve as a resource to the education community by providing information and guidance in the area of access-to-information technologies by individuals with disabilities. <http://easi.cc>

Job Accommodation Network. An international toll-free consulting service that provides information about job accommodations and the employability of people with disabilities. <http://janweb.icdi.wvu.edu>

National Assistive Technology Advocacy Project, sponsored by Neighborhood Legal Services, provides an excellent clearinghouse of information on AT advocacy. <http://www.nls.org/natmain.htm.>

National Center for the Dissemination of Disability Research (NCDDR). Disseminates information about disability research, including assistive technology. <http://www.ncddr.org/>

National Center on Accessibility. An organization committed to the full participation in parks, recreation and tourism by people with disabilities. <http://www.indiana.edu/~nca/nca.htm>

National Clearinghouse of Rehabilitation Training Materials. Funded by the Rehabilitation Services Administration, this site provides an extensive array of disability related training resources. <http://www.nchrtm.okstate.edu/>

National Library of Medicine listing of links related to assistive technology. http://www.nlm.nih.gov/medlineplus/assistivedevices.html

National Rehabilitation Information Center. A library and information center on disability and rehabilitation. <http://www.naric.com/search/at.html>

RESNA's Technical Assistance Project Library. Summarizes key legislation and provides links to resources such as an AT bibliography. http://www.resna.org/taproject/library/

Included is a link to a paper by the Regional Center for Independent Living describing the peer mentor program that created the materials in Appendix B. http://www.resna.org/taproject/library/match.html

International:

Disabled Peoples' International. Searchable by country and very extensive. http://www.dpi.org/en/resources/topics.htm

World Information on Disability site. http://www.sd.soft.iwate-pu.ac.jp/sensui/foreign_res.html

The following are excellent portals for obtaining information about assistive technology in Canada, Europe and Australia:

Canada

http://www.pwd-online.ca/pwdhome.jsp?lang=en

Europe

Central Remedial Clinic, Client Technical Services, Ireland. Describes projects to empower users of assistive technology. http://www.crc.ie/services/technology/projects.htm

EUSTAT- Empowering Users Through Assistive Technology. http://www.siva.it/research/eustat/index.html

Association for the Advancement of Assistive Technology in Europe. http://139.91.151.134/index.asp?auto-redirect=true&accept-initial-profile=standard

Australia

http://www.e-bility.com

Other Recommended Links:

http://www.ablenetinc.com – (teaching children with disabilities)

http://www.icdi.wvu.edu/others.htm – (general)

http://www.spinalcord.uab.edu – (spinal cord injury information)

http://www.infouse.com – (disability statistics and a variety of resources)

http://www.apa.org/divisions/div22 – (bibliography on rehabilitation topics)

http://members.aol.com/IMPT97/MPT.html – (Institute for Matching Person & Technology homepage)

A Sample of Good Reading Available on the Web:

Assistive Technology: Frequently Asked Questions by the Alliance for Technology Access: http://www.ataccess.org/resources/fpic/faq/default.html

Assistive Technology Survey Results: Continued Benefits and Needs Reported by Americans with Disabilities: http://www.ncddr.org/du/researchexchange/v07n01/atpaper/

Funding Assistive Technology and Accommodations by the National Center on Workforce and Disability/Adult: http://www.onestops.info/article.php?article_id=22&subcat_id=3

Informed Consumer's Guide to Funding Assistive Technology by the National Institute on Disability and Rehabilitation Research:
http://www.abledata.com/text2/funding.htm

Make sure the Medical device You Choose is Designed for You by the U.S. Food and Drug Administration Center for Devices and Radiological Health. This web site contains a checklist for health care professionals and patients to use when choosing a medical device that is best for the patient.
http://www.fda.gov/cdrh/humfac/you_choose_checklist.html

Unmet Needs: Statistics on the Lack of Access to Assistive Devices, Technologies and Related Services:
http://www.itemcoalition.org/press/unmet.html

Assistive Technology Device Predisposition Assessment

As professionals strive to keep up with the times, and effectively meet the needs of the people with whom they are working, it is imperative that the individuals who will be using technologies make the choices about what will best assist them. In this way, the chances that the device will actually meet the person's needs are greatly increased. *The Matching Person and Technology* process provides the steps toward acquiring technology that will best meet the needs of the individuals with disabilities by encouraging professionals to thoroughly investigate the milieu or the environments of use, the preferences and characteristics of the individual and the most appropriate features of the technology.

The following is an actual case report where the MPT process was used to inform decisions about the most appropriate interventions for a particular consumer with cerebral palsy. Written by a working rehabilitation professional enrolled in an online masters degree in rehabilitation counseling,* it has been edited from the original to make it more concise and to preserve the anonymity of the individuals involved.

REPORT

I. Description of Focus Individual.

Tim is an existing recipient of services from a community rehabilitation agency and he is now inquiring about devices that could assist him in turning the pages of books. He is quite frustrated with how often he is ruining books by ripping the pages while trying to read

Tim is thirty years old and has always been interested in helping people. He uses a powered wheelchair and a communication device to support him in volunteering four days a week at a local assisted living facility and has dreams of going to school someday for counseling or social work. Tim has openly shared with me in the past his struggles with cerebral palsy, and with depression. He feels that helping others has forced him to keep a good perspective about his own life. Tim has a great memory and enjoys discussions about history. When asked about his interests, he stated that he likes spending time with his girlfriend, learning about history, and eating good food. His roommate, who

*This real case study was initiated for an assignment in the Applications of Rehabilitation Technology course, one of the required courses in an online masters degree in Rehabilitation Counseling offered collaboratively by San Diego State University, University of North Texas, and Georgia State University. Dr. Caren Sax created and teaches the course online for the Consortium and on campus at SDSU.

is paid to provide whatever supports Tim might need to be as independent as possible, added that Tim spends a lot of time watching television, especially the history channel, and using his computer. He added that his main focus lately has been reading a new collection of coffee table style history books that were a gift from his brother.

II. MPT Results & Analysis.

Tim and I started the MPT process with his target activity already in mind. Due to the spasticity and tremors that he experiences in his hands and fingers from his CP, he is unable to control his hands or fingers to manipulate the pages of books without ripping them. His immediate goal is to read his brand new coffee table history book collection without ruining any of them and his long-term goal is to take classes one day without fear that he will be unable to independently read the required books. He hopes to find a device that he can easily incorporate into his lifestyle.

We completed the *Initial Worksheet for the Matching Person & Technology Model* to help us focus in on the area that Tim wanted to target for technology use if we did not already have one in mind. Tim currently uses an electronic communication device, a *Dynavox*, and has used a manual communication board in the past. He went through years of speech therapy and has a negative view of speech pathologists. He uses an electric wheelchair for mobility purposes. His apartment is adapted so that it is quite accessible to him with ramps, lowered counters, grab bars, etc. He effectively uses an eye gaze system for accessing both his communication device and his computer. He seems to feel that he has the adaptive equipment he needs in most areas of his life.

Next, Tim and I completed the consumer version of the *Survey of Technology Use* which reviewed the devices that Tim had tried in the past for a variety of support needs, and revealed Tim's rather negative memories of trying to find devices that he would actually use, particularly communication devices. He shared that he had very little help in his younger years and several negative experiences with AT during his Junior High and High School years. He spoke more positively of recent experiences in finding AT with his current roommate. Tim has explored different medical ways of controlling his spasticity, such as the use of Baclofen, but has not experienced much of an improvement. Tim shared that he had tried a variety of ways to turn the pages of books. His roommate would often help him by standing by and turning the pages when Tim was ready, but then Tim could only read when his roommate was around. They had tried tape on his hands and sticks with tacky substances on the end but all ended unsatisfactorily and, in Tim's words, 'with a mess.' We discussed using books on tape to avoid the turning of pages altogether and the possibility of using the Internet for classes; however, Tim was not very open to those ideas as he said he enjoys the experience of reading and the coffee table books include many pictures that he would miss out on with the audiotapes.

At our next meeting, Tim and I completed two forms: the Assistive Technology Device Predisposition Assessment (ATD PA) - Person and the Assistive Technology Device Predisposition Assessment (ATD PA) – Device. While completing these forms, the questions sparked conversation around topics that Tim and I had never discussed before. I found out a lot about Tim's overall attitude toward trying AT and about his confidence levels. His incentives for using AT included his desire to read books at his leisure, to pursue his hobby of collecting coffee table books about history, to decrease his frustration levels, to increase his success at reading, to decrease his embarrassing moments like when he returns ripped books to the library, to overcome his fears of not being able to read required books for school so that he will pursue his career, and to be a happier person, overall. Some disincentives that came up during our conversations included his fears of not fitting in because of yet another large device to show off his disability, memories of bad experiences about devices that did not do what he thought that they would, and anxiety about not being able to use the device. Although I was surprised at the negativity that surfaced during a lot of our discussion, I still felt pretty confident that one of the electronic page turners was going to be a good match for him when I sent in my ATD PA forms to be scored and interpreted.

As I read through the analysis after it was sent back to me, many of the results caused me to question the success of an electronic page turner. Noteworthy is the fact that Tim saw a lot more limitations than capabilities in himself, had a negative general mood state, showed dissatisfaction with his current well-being/quality of life, and did not seem to feel he had a strong natural support system. In addition, , he demonstrates low self-esteem and may have difficulty exploring undertaking new strategies or new directions at this time and may not be ready to accept a significant new challenge. I started to question my initial optimism about the use of an electronic page turner wondering if it might be too much of a device at this time. I shared the results with Tim who said that he wanted to go ahead with the search for a device and at the same time, give more thought to how he was feeling.

III. Implementation & Recommendations.
Tim and I met to research the possible devices to help with the turning of pages. We found two that looked like they had the features that would meet Tim's needs. As we inspected each item, Tim and I tried to look at both their positive and negative aspect. Tim mentioned several times that the devices were large. For his current need, he wanted to be able to turn the pages of coffee table books and so I had been concentrating on the larger devices and the more high tech devices that could accommodate the size of the books. Tim started looking at smaller devices, particularly a very inexpensive device called a Vacuum Wand that he loved from the looks of it.

As Tim and I discussed all of the options, we talked more about his general feelings about himself and his future. He recognized a lot of his fears and said that when he had gotten his wheelchair and his communication device he felt a lot of the same feelings. He admitted that he had been feeling very anxious about the cost of the electronic devices, and the size of them; however, he was excited and did not want to hurt my feelings as I was so excited about the electronic devices. He said that he already has his *Dynavox*, and his computer and he did not want to have to deal with another bulky item just to read a book. He said that in the future when he looks into classes he might be more open to the electronic device. We had a good "meeting of the minds," and I shared that the only reason we were doing this search was to find something that would work for him, and that while I appreciated his thoughtfulness, I would not be hurt at all if we switched gears and focused more on the smaller items such as the Vacuum Wand. When I asked him if he thought it would be a good idea to speak with his psychologist about his present state of mind, and his high levels of frustration, he said that he thought that would be helpful. He invited his girl-friend to discuss the results of the analysis with us and she suggested also that talking to the psychologist would be a good idea. We followed up with a call to his psychologist who thought that starting with a simple, easy-to-use device would give Tim opportunity for success that would build his confidence levels. In concordance with the results of the ATD PA analysis, she felt that Tim should focus on improving his self-image and his overall wellbeing before introducing any major changes in his life. Tim and I discussed all of the input we had received and decided to review the top three options for AT:

1) The GEWA Page Turner BLV-6 is an electronic page turner which accommodates most textbooks, paperbacks, magazines, newspapers. It is 12"x9" and can hold books that are up to 2" thick, so it would be able to accommodate Tim's coffee table books. It has a rubber roller which can turn pages forward or backward and can be fixed to a wheelchair or stand. It has a handle for transport and can be hooked up to a variety of input controls to meet Tim's needs. It is available through Zygo at www.zygo-usa.com for $3,395.

2) Touch Turner CR is also an electronic page turner; Model CR allows pages to be turned forward and backward. Various switches can be attached for input such as the Sip-N-Puff, Large Target, and Single Lever. Price is $1,030 without any additional switches at www.touchturner.com.

3) The Vacuum Wand is a low tech device similar to a straw with a suction cup on the end that is manipulated by air being blown into or sucked out of the straw. It is an inexpensive alternative to the electronic page turners, and could utilize Tim's abilities well, enabling him to turn the pages of any size book. It would be easily transportable, preventing him from having to cart around yet another bulky AT device. Tim has the money for this device. We found it in a Sammons Preston Catalogue for $34.95, and he has ordered one to be delivered by 6/30/04!

IV. Funding sources.

Tim and I discussed funding in our very first meeting together as his finances are pretty tight. He said that he has a few hundred dollars in savings and is expecting some money from a relative who just passed away. He thought that he would receive around $1,000 but was not sure. Tim has MediCal for insur-ance and was fairly certain that they would not cover the device, although we agreed to look into that option when the time was right. We talked with the Department of Rehabilitation and found that a device could possibly be covered if Tim were going to school or working which might be an option down the road but not at this time. We found that Tim's brother was a member of the Elk's club and that Tim could write a letter requesting financial assistance if it were needed. We also identified a group of businessmen, called "The Good Guys" who apparently assist people financially on an as needed basis. So, Tim and I agreed to determine how much would be needed first, and then work together to write some convincing letters. Since Tim ended up deciding on a very inexpensive device, he used his own resources and I typed up the other resources for him to keep for future reference.

V. Reflection.

The process from beginning to end was a learning one for me. I recognize that I got overzealous and immediately thought that I had found an easy solution with the electronic page turner. Finding out how depressed Tim really seems to be was unexpected for me and how much was brought out by the questions on the MPT helped me to see the whole picture. I learned that it is important to really listen to what is being said; to not jump to conclusions; and that I could easily be one of those people who help someone to get a device that they don't end up using. Unintentional, but devastating! I think that I probably made Tim feel rather uncomfortable by being overly excited at times about a big, expensive AT but once we were able to get things out into the open all seemed to go well. Tim said he was comfortable with the process and that he felt supported and in control.

I feel that Tim and I were able to match his immediate needs. In the future when he is ready, he may go back to exploring the electronic page turner especially if he decides to pursue school and a career in counseling. Tim is scheduled to get his Vacuum Wand at the end of June. At that point, we will determine how well it will meet his needs. Tim and I discovered several web sites with links to tons of AT devices. Just knowing how simple it is to use the web to access AT will be beneficial for future situations.

Next time, I will be sure to listen from the very beginning to hear exactly what the person's expectations are and what their current situations are, and try to keep in mind the milieu, the person and the technology, and learn more about the specifics of the technology before deciding on it!

I believe that we achieved success because we (hopefully) found a device that meets Tim's immediate needs. Tim is scheduled to receive his device by the end of June and is supposed to call me when it arrives. We have a tentative date to get together on 7/1 to see how it works for him. He has set aside the money to pay for it and has his stack of books ready to read! I also assisted Tim in maintaining records of all of the assessments that we completed together and the information on the devices that he decided against for now. In the future, if he decides to pursue an electronic page turner he should have the resources necessary to start his search.

Tim will continue to search for the technology that best meets his needs throughout his life, and working through the MPT process has most likely given him a strong working knowledge of how to go through the process in a timely fashion in the future.

The Matching Person & Technology Assessment Process and Instruments[1]

Step One: *Initial Worksheet for the Matching Person and Technology* (MPT) *Model* is used to determine the consumer's dream, initial goals that the professional and the user have established, including possible alternative goals, and the purpose or task for which the intervention is being considered. Second, potential interventions supportive of these goals are written in the space provided on the form. Third, any technologies needed to support the attainment of the goals are recorded.

Step Two: *History of Support Use* is used to identify technologies used is the past, satisfaction with those technologies, and those which are desired and needed but not yet available to the consumer. The professional and consumer complete this form collaboratively.

Step Three: The consumer is asked to complete his or her version of the appropriate form depending on the type of technology under consideration (general, assistive (see sample in this Appendix), educational, workplace or healthcare).[2] The user form may serve as a guide for an oral interview, if that seems more appropriate for the situation. The professional completes the professional version of the same form and identifies any discrepancies in perspective between the professional's and the consumer's responses. These discrepancies then become a topic for discussion and negotiation.

Step Four: The professional discusses with the user those factors that may indicate problems with his or her acceptance or appropriate use of the technology.

Step Five: After problem areas have been noted, the professional and consumer work to identify specific intervention strategies and devise an action plan to address the problems.

Step Six: The strategies and action plans are committed to writing, for experience has shown that plans that are merely verbalized are not implemented as frequently as written plans. Written plans also serve as documentation and can provide the justification for any subsequent actions such as requests for funding or release time for training.

Step Seven: A follow-up assessment is conducted to determine any adjustments or accommodations needed to the technology and to inquire into goal achievement and whether the consumer has changed priorities.

Footnotes:

[1] The MPT forms have been linked to the World Health Organization's International Classification of Functioning, Disability and Health (ICF) and the ISO9999 standards (assistive technology). You can freely access this article, copy and distribute it, as long as you cite the Newsletter as the source. Here is the citation for the article, with the URL you need to access it:

Scherer, M.J. (2004). Enhancing assistive technology selection and use: Connecting the ICF and ISO9999. Newsletter on the WHO-FIC, 2(1), 10-11.
http://www.rivm.nl/who-fic/newsletter/newsletter2004-1.pdf_

[2] There is a complete manual describing the administration and scoring of each measure, interpretation and use of the results, as well as the reliability and validity of the measures. More information is available at this URL:
http://members.aol.com/IMPT97/MPT.html

Assistive Technology Device Predisposition Assessment

Representative Sample (this sample shows only half of the items)

Name	Date of Birth
Primary Goals (6 months):	Today's Date
Primary Goals (1 year+):	Form completed by

A. How would you rate your abilities today in the following 9 areas using your current AT or other support?

- For items 1-9, circle the best response (1 for *poor* through 5 for *excellent*).
- Under *Name of Support* write the name of the support you use where relevant (example: 'eyeglasses' for # 1, *eyesight*).
- Write a plus [+] in the spaces where you expect to need more support over the next year (example: 'eyeglasses' gets [+] if you'll expect to need stronger lenses during the next year). Write a [-] in the spaces where you expect to need less support, and a [0] where you expect your support should stay the same over the next year.

	Poor	Average	Excellent	Name of Support	Need more [+], less [-], same [0]
1. Eyesight	1 2 3 4 5			_____	____
2. Hearing	1 2 3 4 5			_____	____
7. Grasping and use of fingers	1 2 3 4 5			_____	____
9. Mobility	1 2 3 4 5			_____	____

B. How satisfied are you currently in the following areas?

- For items 10 – 21, circle the best response (1 for *Not Satisfied* through 5 for *Very Satisfied*).
- Under *Importance* write #1, #2 or #3 for your three most important areas (#1=most important). Leave the other lines blank.
- Under *Primary Obstacle* write an [E] or [PR] to indicate if the primary obstacle you face is due to external, environmental and social barriers [E] or to limitations you experience due to inadequate AT and other personal resources [PR].

	Not Satisfied	Satisfied	Very Satisfied	Importance	Primary Obstacle [E], [PR]
10. Social relationships	1 2 3 4 5			____	____
15. Recreational involvement	1 2 3 4 5			____	____
16. Freedom to go wherever desired	1 2 3 4 5			____	____
17. Educational attainment	1 2 3 4 5			____	____
20. Autonomy and independence	1 2 3 4 5			____	____
21. Fitting in and belonging	1 2 3 4 5			____	____

C. Please circle all the statements below that describe you.

22. I have the support I want from family
33. I am a calm person
44. I find technology interesting

23. I have the support I want from friends
34. I am patient & easy-going
45. I am cooperative

24. I feel the general public accepts me
36. I am often angry
47. I often feel isolated & alone

26. I am often frustrated or overwhelmed
41. I like having a challenge
52. I often feel insecure

27. I am curious & excited about new things
42. I am satisfied with my life
53. I feel as if I have little privacy

For Comparing Devices to Meet Desired Outcomes

DIRECTIONS: Read each of the twelve items below (A-L) and circle the letter of the *three* that are most important to you.

A. The assistance and accommodations exist for successful use of this device.
B. This device will physically fit in all desired environments (car, living room, etc.).
D. I will benefit from using this device.
G. This device will improve my quality of life.
H. I have the capabilities and stamina to use this device without discomfort, stress and fatigue.
L. I will feel comfortable (and not self conscious) using this device around the community.

Write the name of each device being considered in the boxes below under *Device*. Rate each device for the twelve items (A-L) according to the following scale and then write your ratings in the appropriate boxes:

5 = All the time
4 = Often
3 = Half the time, neutral
2 = Sometimes
1 = Not at all
0 = Not applicable

DEVICE	A	B	C	D	E	F	G	H	I	J	K	L	Total (Add A-L)

Review each **total score**. In general, the device with the highest total score is the one most preferred (maximum number of points=60). However, when total scores are close, more weight should be given to the three items circled as being *most important*.

References

Advance Data From Vital and Health Statistics , No. 292. "Trends and Differential Use of Assistive Technology Devices: United States, 1994.

American Spinal Cord Injury Association. (1996). *International Standards for Neurological and Functional Classification of Spinal Cord Injury.* Revised Edition. Chicago: author.

Basford, J.R., Rohe D.E. & DePompolo, R.W. (2003). Rehabilitation unit staff attitudes toward substance abuse: Changes and similarities between 1985 and 2001. *Archives of Physical Medicine and Rehabilitation,* 84, 1301-7.

Baum, D.D. (1982). *The human side of exceptionality.* Baltimore: University Park Press.

Bennet, J. (April 12, 1992). Wave of sympathy for canine victim. *The New York Times.*

Benshoff, J.J., Janikowski, T.P., Taricone, P.F., & Brenner, J.S. (1990). Alcohol and drug abuse: A content analysis of the rehabilitation literature. *Journal of Applied Rehabilitation Counseling,* 21(4), 9-12.

Bjorck-Akesson, E. (1990, August). *Communicative interaction of young non-speaking children and their parents.* Paper presented at The Fourth Biennial International ISAAC Conference on Augmentative and Alternative Communication, Stockholm, Sweden.

Brightman, A.J. (1984). *Ordinary moments: The disabled experience.* University Park Press.

Brooks, N, & Redden, M.R. (1986). Scientists and engineers with disabilities evaluate assistive devices. *Proceedings of the RESNA 9th Annual Conference* (pp. 1-2). Washington, DC: RESNA.

Brown, D.L. (1996). Personal implications of functional electrical stimulation standing for older adolescents with spinal cord injuries. *Technology & Disability,* 5(3,4), 295-311.

Butt, L. (9 September, 2004). A dignified death: Treatment withdrawal in a person with ventilator-dependent tetraplegia. Presentation for the American Paraplegia Society 50th Annual Conference, September 7-9, Las Vegas.

Carlson, D., Ehrlich, N., Berland, B.J., and Bailey, N., *Assistive Technology Survey Results: Continued Benefits and Needs Reported by Americans with Disabilities,* National Institute on Disability and Rehabilitation Research, 2001.

Condeluci, A. (1989). Empowering people with cerebral palsy. *Journal of Rehabilitation,* 55(2), 15-16.

Consortium for Spinal Cord Medicine. (1999). *Outcomes Following Traumatic Spinal Cord Injury: Clinical Practice Guidelines for Health-Care Professionals.* Washington, DC: Paralyzed Veterans of America.

Creech, R. (1990, August). Practical augmentative and alternative communication: The ultimate goal. Paper presented at The Fourth Biennial International ISAAC Conference on Augmentative and Alternative Communication, Stockholm, Sweden.

Crewe, N. and Dijkers, M. (1995). Functional assessment. In L.A. Cushman & M.J. Scherer (eds). *Psychological Assessment in Medical Rehabilitation* (pp.101-144). Washington, DC: APA Books.

Cushman, L.A. & Scherer, M.J. (1998). Perceived needs and person-technology fit in spinal cord injury. *Conference Program of the 12th Annual Conference of the American Association of Spinal Cord Injury Psychologists and Social Workers*, 28-29.

DeVivo, M.J., Jackson, A., Dijkers, M. & Poczatek, R. (9 September, 2004). Etiology of spinal cord injury: Trends over three decades. Presentation for the American Paraplegia Society 50th Annual Conference, September 7-9, Las Vegas.

Dijkers M. (1997). Quality of life after spinal cord injury: A meta analysis of the effects of disablement components. *Spinal Cord*, 35(12), 829-40.

Dragona, J.J. (1985/2). The joys of advocacy: Will we ever be permitted to rest upon our laurels? *Disabled USA*, 34-35.

Dudek, R.A. (1985). *Human rehabilitation techniques: A technology assessment.* Paper presented at the national meeting of the American Hospital Association, New Orleans. (NARIC Document No. R002672).

Elliott, T.R. & Umlauf, R.L. (1995). Measurement of personality and psychopathology following acquired physical disability. In L.A. Cushman & M.J. Scherer (eds). *Psychological Assessment in Medical Rehabilitation* (pp. 325-358). Washington, DC: APA Books.

Enders, A. (1984). Questionable devices. *Proceedings of the Second Annual Meeting of the Rehabilitation Engineering Society of North America* (pp. 271-276). Bethesda, MD: Rehabilitation Engineering Society of North America (RESNA).

Evans, R.W., Manninen, D.L., Garrison, L.P., Hart, L.G., Blagg, C.R., Gutman, R.A., Hull, A.R., & Lowrie, e.g., (1985). The quality of life of patients with end-stage renal disease. *New England Journal of Medicine*, 312(9), 553-559.

Gage, N.L., & Berliner, D.C. (1992). *Educational Psychology,* Fifth Edition. Boston: Houghton Mifflin.

Galvin, J.C., & Scherer, M.J. (eds.). (1996). *Evaluating, selecting, and using appropriate assistive technology.* Gaithersburg, MD: Aspen Publishers, Inc.

Garris, A.G. (1983/3). Is it righteous or outrageous: Responses to thoughts on rage and disability. *Disabled USA*, 10.

Greer, B.G. (1986). Substance abuse among people with disabilities: A problem of too much accessibility. *Journal of Rehabilitation*, 52(1), 34-38.

Gilligan, C. (1982). *In a different voice: Psychological theory and women's development.* Cambridge, Mass.: Harvard University Press.

Hansell, N. (1974). *The person-in-distress: On the biosocial mechanisms of adaptation.* New York: Behavioral Sciences Press.

Harris, L., & Associates. (1991). *Public attitudes toward people with disabilities.* National Council on Disability. Washington, DC.

Heinemann, A.W. (1991). *Substance abuse and spinal cord injury.* Paraplegia News, 45(7), 16.

Kaplan, S., & Questad, K. (1980). Client characteristics in rehabilitation studies: A literature review. *Journal of Applied Rehabilitation Counseling,* 11(4), 165-168.

Klebine, P. and Lindsey, L. (2000). Sexual function for men with spinal cord injury. Spinal Cord Injury Information Network: Rehabilitation Research and Training Center on Secondary Conditions of SCI and Model SCI Care Center. University of Alabama at Birmingham Spain Rehabilitation Center.

Kottke, F.J. (1982). Philosophic considerations of quality of life for the disabled. *Archives of Physical Medicine and Rehabilitation,* 63, 60-62.

Krause, J.S. (1999). Correlates of depression after spinal cord injury: Incidence, correlates, case studies, and treatment. *Conference Program of the 13th Annual Conference of the American Association of Spinal Cord Injury Psychologists and Social Workers,* 22.

Krause, J.S., Crewe, N.M. & Kemp, B.J. (1999). Depression among individuals living in the community with spinal cord injury: Incidence, correlates, case studies, and treatment. Conference Program of the 13th *Annual Conference of the American Association of Spinal Cord Injury Psychologists and Social Workers,* 22.

Krause, J.S., & Crewe, N.M. (1987). Prediction of long-term survival among persons with spinal cord injury: An 11-year prospective study. *Rehabilitation Psychology,* 32, 205-213.

Krause, J.S., DeVivo, M., Jackson, A., Pickelsimer, E. & Broderick, L. (2004). Risk factors for mortality after spinal cord injury [abstract]. *Archives of Physical Medicine and Rehabilitation,* 85(8), E1.

Kubler-Ross, E. (1969). *On death and dying.* New York: Macmillan.

Kutner, B. (1969). Professional antitherapy. *Journal of Rehabilitation,* 35(6), 16-18.

Lammertse, D.P. (1999). Restorative research in spinal cord injury: A rehabilitationist's perspective. *Conference Program of the 13th Annual Conference of the American Association of Spinal Cord Injury Psychologists and Social Workers,* 23.

Lange, M.L. (1995). Aiming high. *TeamRehab Report.* 6(9), 26-30.

LaPlante, M.P., Hendershot, G.E., & Moss, A.J. (September 16, 1992). *Assistive technology devices and home accessibility features: Prevalence, payment, need, and trends.* Advance Data (National Center for Health Statistics), No. 217.

Lassiter, R.A. (1972). History of the rehabilitation movement in America. In Cull, J.G., & Hardy, R.E. (Eds.), *Vocational rehabilitation: Profession and process.* Springfield, IL: Charles C. Thomas.

Lathrop, D. (1997, April). Remember 504. *Mainstream,* 32-34.

Lindsey, L. Klebine, P. and Wells, M.J. (2000). *Understanding SCI and Functional Goals.* Spinal Cord Injury Information Network: Rehabilitation Research and

Training Center on Secondary Conditions of SCI and Model SCI Care Center. University of Alabama at Birmingham Spain Rehabilitation Center.

Littrell, J.L. (1991). Women with disabilities in community college computer training programs. In H. Murphy (Ed.), *Proceedings of the Sixth Annual Conference, Technology and Persons with Disabilities* (pp. 553-562), California State University, Northridge.

Maslow, A.H. 1954). *Motivation and personality*. New York: Harper & Row.

Maynard, F.M., & Muth, A.S. (1987). The choice to end life as a ventilator-dependent quadriplegic. *Archives of Physical Medicine & Rehabilitation*, 68(12), 862-864.

McColl, M.A., Bickenbach, J., Johnston, J., Nishihama, S., Schumaker, M., Smith, K., Smith, M. & Yealland, B. (2000). Changes in spiritual beliefs after traumatic disability. *Archives of Physical Medicine & Rehabilitation*, 81, 817-823.

Musselwhite, C.R. (1990, August). *Topic setting: Generic and specific strategies*. Paper presented at The Fourth Biennial International ISAAC Conference on Augmentative and Alternative Communication, Stockholm, Sweden.

National Council on Disability. (1996). *Achieving independence: The challenges for the 21st century*. Washington, DC: Author.

National Council on Disability. (1998, July). New NOD/Harris Survey of Americans with Disabilities. *NCD Bulletin*. Washington, DC: Author.

New York State Senate Select Committee on the Disabled, L. Paul Kehoe, Chairman. (1989). *Coming to terms with disabilities: A compilation of vocabulary relating to visible and non-visible disabilities*. Albany, New York: Author.

Nolan, C. (1987). *Under the eye of the clock: The life story of Christopher Nolan*. New York: St. Martin's Press.

Nosek, M.A. (1990). Personal assistance: Key to employability of persons with physical disabilities. *Journal of Applied Rehabilitation Counseling*, 21(4), 3-8.

Nosek, M.A., Fuhrer, M.J., & Potter, C. (1995). Life satisfaction of people with physical disabilities: Relationship to personal assistance, disability status, and handicap. *Rehabilitation Psychology*, 40(3), 191-202.

Novack, T.A. & Gage, R.J. (1995). Assessment of family functioning and social support. In L.A. Cushman & M.J. Scherer (eds). *Psychological Assessment in Medical Rehabilitation* (pp.275-297). Washington, DC: APA Books.

Parette, H.P., Huer, M.B. & Scherer, M. (2004). Effects of acculturation on assistive technology service delivery. *Journal of Special Education Technology*, 19(2), 31-41.

Perkes, D. (1995). Rusk, Howard A. In A.E. Dell Orto & R.P. Marinelli (Eds.), Encyclopedia of disability and rehabilitation (pp. 651-652). New York: Macmillan Library Reference USA.

Phillips, B., & Zhao, H. (1993). Predictors of assistive technology abandonment. *Assistive Technology*, 5, 36-45.

Rahimi, M.A. (1981/January). Intelligent prosthetic devices. *Computer*, p. 22.

Richardson, S.J., & Poulson, D.F. (1994). Requirements capture in rehabilitation ergonomics. IEA '94. *Proceedings of the 12th Triennial Congress of the International Ergonomics Association*. Vol. 3, 15-19 *August* 1994, *Toronto, Canada*, pp. 16-18.

Richmond, G. (1996, March). Living independently using assistive technology: A dollars and sense approach. *Tapping Technology (Maryland Technology Assistance Program)*, 1-2.

Rintala D.H., Herson, L. & Hudler-Hull, T. (1999). Comparison of parenting styles and children's outcomes between parents with and without a spinal cord injury. *Conference Program of the 13th Annual Conference of the American Association of Spinal Cord Injury Psychologists and Social Workers*, 25.

Roessler, R.T. (1990). A quality of life perspective on rehabilitation counseling. *Rehabilitation Counseling Bulletin*, 34(2), 82-90.

Rohe, D.E., & DePompolo, R.W. (1985). Substance abuse policies in rehabilitation medicine departments. *Archives of Physical Medicine & Rehabilitation*, 66, 701-703.

Rohe, D.E., & Krause, J.S. (1992, August). *Stability of interests after severe physical disability: An 11-year longitudinal study*. Paper presented at the 100th Annual Meeting of the American Psychological Association, Washington, D.C.

Root, A.A. (1970). What instructors say to the students makes a difference. *Engineering Education*, 61, 722-725.

Rosen, S.L. (1983). Learning to be handicapped. *Disabled USA*, (1), 7-9.

Rush, W.L. (1985). Not a fifth wheel: Sexual expression needs to be main-streamed, too. *Disabled USA*, 2, 26-29.

Scherer, M.J. (1998, Revision of 1991 Edition). *The Matching Person & Technology (MPT) Model Manual and accompanying assessment instruments*. Webster, NY: Author. [http://members.aol.com/IMPT97/MPT.html]

Scherer, M.J. (1984). *A descriptive study of regional spinal cord injured data bases with special emphasis on selected variables in the base managed by Strong Memorial Hospital*. Unpublished paper, University of Rochester School of Medicine and Dentistry, Department of Preventive, Family, and Rehabilitation Medicine.

Scherer, M.J. (1988a). Assistive device utilization and quality of life in adults with spinal cord injuries or cerebral palsy. *Journal of Applied Rehabilitation Counseling*, 19(2), 21-30.

Scherer, M.J. (1988b). Differing perspectives of the use of assistive technology devices (ATDs) by people with physical disabilities. In H. Murphy (Ed.), *Proceedings of the Fourth Annual Conference, "Technology and Persons with Disabilities"* (pp. 444-453). Los Angeles: Office of Disabled Student Services, California State University, Northridge.

Scherer, M.J. (1990). Assistive device utilization and quality of life in adults with spinal cord injuries or cerebral palsy: Two years later. *Journal of Applied Rehabilitation Counseling*, 21(4), 36-44.

Scherer, M.J. (1991a). Assistive technology use, avoidance and abandonment: What we know so far. In H. Murphy (Ed.), *Proceedings of the Sixth Annual Conference, Technology and Persons with Disabilities* (pp. 815-826), California State University, Northridge.

Scherer, M.J. (1991b). *Psychosocial factors associated with women's use of technological assistance.* Paper presented at the 99th annual convention of the American Psychological Association, San Francisco. (Cassette Recording No. APA-91-306).

Scherer, M.J. (2002). The change in emphasis from people to person: introduction to the special issue on Assistive Technology. *Disability & Rehabilitation,* 24(1/2/3), 1-4.

Scherer, M.J. & Craddock, G. (2002). Matching Person & Technology (MPT) assessment process. *Technology & Disability, Special Issue: The Assessment of Assistive Technology Outcomes, Effects and Costs,* 14(3), 125-131.

Scherer, M.J. & Frisina, D.R. (1998). Characteristics associated with marginal hearing loss and subjective well-being among a sample of older adults. *Journal of Rehabilitation Research and Development,* 35(4), 420-426.

Scofield, G.R. (1999). Decisions about the end of life. *American Association of Spinal Cord Injury Psychologists and Social Workers (AASCIPSW) 1999 Conference Program and Abstracts,* page 28. Jackson Heights, NY: AASCIPSW.

Scott, R.A. (1969). *The making of blind men: A study of adult socialization.* New York: Russell Sage Foundation.

Skow, J. (August 17, 1987). Heroism, hugs and laughter. *Time,* 60.

Smith, Q.W., Frieden, L., & Richards, L. (1995). Independent living. In A.E. Dell Orto & R.P. Marinelli (Eds.), *Encyclopedia of disability and rehabilitation* (pp. 399-406). New York: Macmillan.

Spinal cord injury facts and figures at a glance. (2003). Spinal Cord Injury Information Network: Rehabilitation Research and Training Center on Secondary Conditions of SCI and Model SCI Care Center. University of Alabama at Birmingham Spain Rehabilitation Center.

Starkey, P.D. (1967). Sick role retention as a factor in nonrehabilitation. *Journal of Counseling Psychology,* 15(1), 75-79.

Sternberg, R. (2003, May. Presidents column: the other three R's: part three, resilience. *Monitor on Psychology,* 34(5), 5.

Stinson, M.S., Scherer, M. J., & Walter, G. G. (1988). Factors affecting persistence of deaf college students. *Research in Higher Education,* 27(3), 244-258.

Stoll, K. (1983/1). Laughter is part of a survivor's handbook. *Disabled USA,* 10-12.

Sullivan, M. (1926). *Our times: The turn of the century.* New York: Charles Scribner's Sons.

Szalai, A., & Andrews, F.M. (1980). *The quality of life: Comparative studies.* Beverly Hills, CA: Sage Publications, Inc.

The University of Alabama National Spinal Cord Injury Statistical Center, Centers for Disease Control and Prevention, 2003.

Thomason, T.C. (1990). Assistive technology for rural American Indians. In H. Murphy (Ed.), *Proceedings of the Fifth Annual Conference, "Technology and Persons with Disabilities"* (pp. 695-701). Los Angeles: Office of Disabled Student Services, California State University, Northridge.

Trieschmann, R.B. (1988). *Spinal cord injuries: Psychological, social, and vocational rehabilitation* (2nd ed.). New York: Demos Publications.

Ulicny, G.R., White, G.W., Bradford, B., & Mathews, R.M. (1990). Consumer exploitation by attendants: How often does it happen and can anything be done about it? *Rehabilitation Counseling Bulletin, 33*(3), 240-246.

United States Census Bureau, Americans with disabilities, 2000.

U.S. National Center for Health Statistics. (1994). Trends and Differential Use of Assistive Technology Devices: United States, 1994. Retrieved August 12, 2004, from http://www.cdc.gov/nchs/.

Vash, C.L. (1981). *The psychology of disability*. New York: Springer Publishing Co.

Welch, R.D., Lobley, S.J., O'Sullivan, S.B., & Freed, M.M. (1986). Functional independence in quadriplegia: Critical levels. *Archives of Physical Medicine & Rehabilitation, 67*, 235-240.

Whitbourne, S.K. (2004). *The aging individual: Physical and psychological perspectives*. New York: Springer Publishing Company.

Whiteneck, G.G., Charlifue, S.W., Frankel, H.L., Fraser, M.H., Gardner, B.P., Gerhart, K.A., Krishnan, K.R., Menter, R.R., Nuseibeh, I., Short, D.J., & Silver, J.R. (1992). Mortality, morbidity, and psychosocial outcomes of persons spinal cord injured more than 20 years ago. *Paraplegia, 30*, 617-630.

Whyte, W.F. (Ed.). (1991). *Participatory action research*. Newbury Park, CA: Sage Publications, Inc.

Willmuth, M.E. & Holcomb, L. (Eds.). (1993). *Women with disabilities: Found voices*. New York: The Haworth Press, Inc.

Wright, B.A. (1960). *Physical disability: A psychological approach.* New York: Harper & Row.

Yarkony, G.M., & Chen, D. (1996). Rehabilitation of patients with spinal cord injuries. In R.L. Braddon (Ed.), *Physical medicine and rehabilitation* (pp. 1149-1179). Philadelphia: W.B. Saunders Co.

Zapf, S.A. (1998a). *The Analysis of the Service Animal Adaptive Intervention Assessment.* Unpublished master's thesis, Texas Woman's University, Denton, TX.

Zapf, S.A. (1998b). *Service Animal Adaptive Intervention Assessment (SAAIA): A Process and Series of Assessments for Evaluating Predispositions to and Outcomes of Service Animal Use.* Webster, NY: The Institute for Matching Person & Technology, Inc. [http:members.aol.com/IMPT97/MPT.html].

Zola, I.K. (1984). Disincentives to independent living. In *Proceedings of the 2nd International Conference on Rehabilitation Engineering* (pp. 121-125), Washington, D.C.: RESNA Press.

A

abandonment of devices, ii, xiii, xiv, xvii, 117–119, 139, 182
reasons for, 118
accessibility, 50, 77, 138, 141, 152, 154, 183
accomplishment, 74, 76, 78, 82, 85,
. See also achievement
achievement, 74, 85, 96–99, 107, 114, 115, 126, 128, 131, 184. See also accomplishment
activities of daily living (ADL), 40, 42, 44
adapted equipment, 16, 21, 37
aging, 92, 94, 128, 170
alcohol. See substance abuse
American Coalition of Citizens with Disabilities, vii
Americans with Disabilities Act (ADA), ix, 40, 45, 51, 54, 75, 152, 154, 178, 183
anger, 2, 11, 97, 99, 106, 108, 171, 172
Ann, 87–92, 128, 169–170
anxiety, 88, 97, 99, 112, 127, 128
augmentative communication, 33, 34, 35
autonomy, xi, 66, 76, 78, 85, 137-138
Axelson, Peter, xi, xii

B

Baum, 1982, 26
Bennet, 1992, 69
Benshoff, Janikowski, Taricone, & Brenner, 1990, 108
Bjorck-Akesson, 1990, 125
Blissymbolics, 29
Bouvia, Elizabeth, 86
Bowe, Frank, vii, x
Brian, 11–16, 18, 19–20, 27–28, 38, 45, 58, 62, 64, 72, 79–81, 105, 111, 132, 145–151, 154
Brightman, 1984, 64
Brown, 1996, 141
Butch, xiii, 59–65, 69, 71, 72, 79, 111–113, 115, 130, 152–154, 170–171, 172, 176, 178

C

cancer, 156, 170
canes, 40, 42
Chris, 55–59, 62, 64, 71, 74, 110, 130, 151, 163, 173, 175, 176
Chuck, 1-4, 5, 9, 10, 11, 16–19, 20, 27–28, 38, 45, 51, 65, 66, 72, 79, 94, 105, 120, 124, 129, 130, 132, 152, 172, 176
civil rights, 31, 49, 54
Civil Rights Act (1964), 49
Civil War, 46
classification of assistive devices
according to environment of use, 41
according to purpose for use, 39–41
according to the functional limitations they address, 41–44

About the Author

Marcia J. Scherer, Ph.D., MPH, FACRM is Director, Institute for Matching Person and Technology <http://members.aol.com/IMPT97/MPT.html>. She is also Senior Research Associate, International Center for Hearing and Speech Research, a joint program of the University of Rochester Medical Center and the National Technical Institute for the Deaf/Rochester Institute of Technology. Additionally, she is Associate Professor of Physical Medicine and Rehabilitation, University of Rochester Medical Center.

Dr. Scherer co-edited (with Jan Galvin) the book *Evaluating, Selecting, and Using Appropriate Assistive Technology* (1996, Aspen Publishers). She also co-edited (with Laura Cushman) the book *Psychological Assessment in Medical Rehabilitation* (1995, American Psychological Association Books) which is Vol. 1 in APA's series "Measurement and Instrumentation in Psychology." She has been honored with fellow status in the American Psychological Association as well as the American Congress of Rehabilitation Medicine. Dr. Scherer is a member of the American Association of Spinal Cord Injury Psychologists and Social Workers, Rehabilitation Engineering and Assistive Technology Society of North America. (RESNA), Australian Rehabilitation & Assistive Technology Association (ARATA), Association for the Advancement of Assistive Technology in Europe (AAATE), the Council for Exceptional Children, and the New York Academy of Sciences.

Dr. Scherer is an alumnus of the S.I. Newhouse School of Public Communications, Syracuse University. She is a Certified Rehabilitation Counselor, and received a master's degree in rehabilitation counseling from the University at Buffalo. Her Ph.D. and MPH degrees are from the University of Rochester. Dr. Scherer is Clinical Associate of the American Board of Medical Psychotherapists.